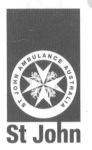

St John

Australian
First Aid

An authorised manual of St John Ambulance Australia

St John Ambulance Australia
Canberra Avenue
Forrest ACT 2603

© St John Ambulance Australia 2006

First edition 1984
Reprinted with corrections 1984–1988
Second edition completely rewritten 1989
Reprinted with corrections 1990–1998
Third edition completely rewritten 1998
Reprinted with corrections 1999–2006
Fourth edition completely rewritten 2006
Reprinted with corrections 3/2007, 8/2007, 4/2008

ISBN 0 949569 55 0

Editor: Shirley Dyson
Design: Goro Jankulovski
Production management: Shirley Dyson
Proofreading: Helen Topor
Typeset in Palatino
Print management: Print Aviator

FOREWORD

Congratulations on receiving your copy of *Australian First Aid*.
In addition, if you have received this book while attending a
St John first aid course, I commend you on your decision to gain
a qualification in first aid.

Knowledge and skills in first aid are essential since unexpected
emergencies can occur without warning. Ideally, we should all
possess the skills, knowledge and confidence to help another person
in need, and possibly to save a life. A first aid emergency may involve
a stranger, but it is more likely that it will be a family member or
a close friend who may need your assistance.

Australian First Aid is the comprehensive authorised manual of
St John Ambulance Australia for first aid training. It represents the
culmination of over 100 years teaching and practice of first aid and
resuscitation by St John in Australia. This information comprises the
latest knowledge from research as reviewed by St John experts and
consultants, in association with relevant international and Australian
professional first aid bodies such as the Australian Resuscitation
Council.

The book is designed for Australian conditions, and contains
clear and simple first aid advice and techniques for any emergency.
The first chapter is *A quick guide to first aid*. This is followed by a series
of colour-coded chapters covering most commonly encountered
injuries and illnesses.

With your up-to-date copy of *Australian First Aid*, a well stocked first
kit and the relevant first aid training, I know that you will be able
to deal more confidently and render first aid more effectively to
someone suffering an emergency—from a blood nose to a bee sting,
or a sudden illness such as chest pain or an allergic reaction.

I trust that this completely authoritative text of St John will become
your principal reference for first aid in your workplace or home.

Dr Peter Warfe, CSC, CStJ
Director of Training
St John Ambulance Australia

Contents

St John 'Caring for life in the community'

St John is a self-funding charitable organisation active throughout the Australian community, dedicated to helping people in sickness, distress, suffering or danger.

Our network of experienced and professional volunteers, together with our paid members, deliver a high level service to the community, supported predominantly by funds raised through the sale of first aid training courses and products.

St John, as a Registered Training Organisation, is Australia's leading first aid training provider. Each year, St John trains over 300,000 people in practical life-saving skills.

Our courses combine theory with 'hands-on' scenario-based training, giving you the skills and confidence to know what to do in an emergency. After completing the Senior First Aid course, why not choose from our contemporary range of courses. To maintain your skill level and stay informed of any changes in first aid, it is important to update your skills regularly.

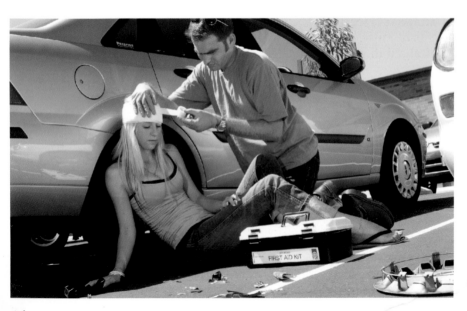

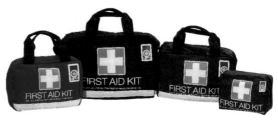

St John first aid kits and equipment

St John has a range of first aid kits designed to manage injuries commonly sustained in the home, at leisure, on the road or in the workplace. Our workplace first aid kits are designed to meet all workplace Occupational Health and Safety (OH&S) requirements. Always remember to check the contents and expiry dates of items in your kit to ensure that you are always ready.

St John volunteers at work

St John volunteers are trained to a professional level to provide high quality first aid care at public events throughout Australia and to manage a diverse range of community care and support programs.

Our volunteer first aiders, distinctive in their black and white uniforms, or outfitted in green overalls provide first aid services at events ranging from local fairs and large and small sporting events to music festivals. St John also provides support during local and national emergencies and disasters.

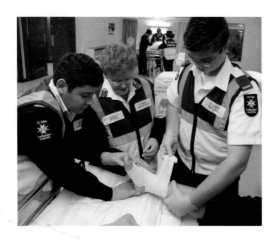

Our Community Care volunteers render care and support to those in need of special help. Programs focus on those in the community experiencing difficulties because of age, disability, isolation, educational limitations or other factors restricting their capacity to lead a normal life.

St John offers a national youth development program for volunteers as young as 8 years. These young members engage in a range of interest and proficiency courses and have the opportunity to develop their leadership and life-saving skills.

St John cadets receive ongoing training so they can participate in various first aid duties under adult supervision. Many have found this early first aid training to be invaluable when pursuing a career in medicine.

By joining St John you will meet, work and share in the team spirit with other first aid and community care members.

To register for first aid training, purchase a first aid kit and equipment, become a St John volunteer or make a donation.

Contact St John on 1300 360 455 or visit www.stjohn.org.au

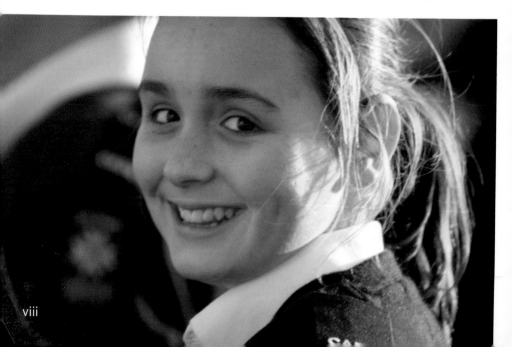

Acknowledgments

St John Ambulance Australia would like to thank all those who have contributed to the development of this fourth edition of Australian First Aid. In particular, the organisation thanks the following groups and individuals for their support:

Members of the Medical Advisory Panel—Dr Peter Warfe, CSC, Professor John Pearn, AM, RFD, Dr Harry Oxer, ASM, Mr Finlay Macneil, Professor Peter Fricker, Professor Paul Arbon, AM, Lt. Col. Geoff Newman-Martin, CSM, RFD.

St John Ambulance – State and Territory Training Branch.

Associate Professor John F. Leditschke, AM, Dr Joan Faoagali, Dr Peter Sullivan, Wayne Deakes, Alan Eade, David Czerkies, Sue Hurdle, Dirk Sunley, Dr William Glasson, Dr Jason Acworth, Dr Peter Sharwood, RFD., Steve Johnson, Russell Dippy, Chris Huggins, Kathryn Zeitz, Chris Bulloch, Dr Elizabeth Gallagher, Margaret Kentler, Robyn Betts, Professor Jeffrey Rosenfeld, Roxy Cowie, OAM, Bob Kearns, David Moss, Terry Jongen, Robert Correa, Jenn Eaton, Peter Barraket, Annetta Albanese, Carol Cunningham (National Heart Foundation of Australia), Maria Said (National President, Anaphylaxis Australia Inc.), Dr Lisa-ann Gershwin (National Marine Stinger Advisor, Surf Life Saving Australia), Christine Barber, Stuart Barber, Molley Barber, Rachael Dyson, Mahala Dyson-Clarke, Maddison Black, Dean Adams, Rachel Lewis, Michael Ray, Susan Fayers, Scott Mitchell, Ron Jacobs, Lucas Perri, Michael Georgiou, Jane Wilson.

Epilepsy Australia
Diabetes Australia
National Asthma Council Australia
National Heart Foundation of Australia
National Stroke Foundation
Anaphylaxis Australia Inc.
Surf Life Saving Australia

St John Ambulance Australia would also like to thank the following organisations for supplying photographic material:

Emergency Management Australia (ref: p. 456)
Australian Capital Territory Ambulance Service (ref: p. 52, 457)
CSIRO Entomology – red-back spider, bee, wasp (ref: p. 343, 345)
Australian Lifesaving Academy, Queensland – cone shell ref: p. 354)
Clay Bryce and the Western Australian Museum – bluebottle (ref: p. 352)
Dr Lisa-ann Gershwin (National Marine Stinger Advisor, Surf Life Saving Australia) – box jellyfish management, Irukandji, blue-ringed octopus (ref: p. 351, 353, 354). Peter Mirtschin – common brown snake (ref: p. 340).

About this book

This St John Ambulance Australia *Australian First Aid* is an authorised manual primarily provided to accompany St John first aid certificate courses. It may also be read as a comprehensive guide to the normal range of first aid procedures, or used as a reference as occasion may demand. It must be stressed, however, that reading this book without attending a St John course with its practical components does not constitute a complete first aid education.

The first chapter—*A quick guide to first aid*—provides the essentials of first aid for the major emergencies a first aider may need to deal with. This ready-reference summary does not substitute for the full coverage given in the main body of the text.

Each chapter begins with an opening page listing the contents included in that chapter.

Throughout the book you will find boxes shaded in green to guide you through first aid management protocols to handle the injury or illness.

An index and glossary are included at the end of the book to assist you.

Emergency telephone numbers

Ambulance, Fire, Police	000 (free call)
Poisons Information Centres	13 11 26
Diver Emergency Service (DES)	1800 088 200
Aust. Venom Research Unit (24 hr)	(03) 8344 7753

1

A quick guide to first aid

DANGER   RESPONSE   AIRWAY

HANDLING AN EMERGENCY

Step 1
ASSESS THE SCENE

Step 2
ASSESS CASUALTY

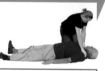

Step 3
OPEN AND CLEAR AIRWAY

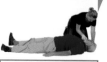

Is there a danger to yourself, others or casualty?

IF **YES**

IF **NO** GO TO **Step 2**

If safe, remove danger OR remove casualty from danger.

Then go to Step 2

Ask casualty for their name, gently squeeze casualty's shoulders.

Is casualty conscious?

IF **NO**

Ask someone to ☎ Call 000 for an ambulance.

Then go to Step 3

IF **YES**

Calm the casualty, monitor signs of life.
Treat any life-threatening injuries.

Open mouth and check for foreign material.

Is there foreign material present?

IF **NO**

Leave on back, open airway.

Then go to Step 4

IF **YES**

Place in recovery position.
Open and clear airway.

Then go to Step 4

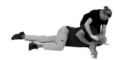

BREATHING	CPR	DEFIBRILLATION

Step 4

CHECK BREATHING

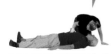

Tilt head back.

Look, listen and feel for breathing, up to 10 seconds.

Is casualty breathing?

IF
NO

Ensure ambulance has been called. If alone with casualty, place in recovery position before calling the ambulance.

Then go to Step 5

IF
YES

Place casualty in recovery position.
☎ *Call 000 for an ambulance*. Monitor signs of life, manage injuries and shock while waiting for ambulance.

Step 5

GIVE INITIAL BREATHS

Turn casualty onto back, give two initial breaths. Ensure chest rises with each breath.

Has breathing returned?

IF
YES

IF
NO
Start CPR.
GO TO
Step 6

Place casualty in recovery position; check regularly for continued signs of life.

Manage any injuries and shock until medical aid arrives.

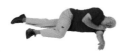

Step 6

PERFORM CPR

Give 30 compressions on lower half of breastbone, then tilt head, lift chin and give 2 breaths.

Alternate 30 compressions with 2 breaths until medical aid arrives.

ADULT/CHILD compressions— use two hands with fingers interlocked.

INFANT compressions— use two fingers.

Stop CPR if casualty shows signs of life, ambulance arrives or you are physically unable to continue.

Step 7

APPLY DEFIBRILLATOR

If a defibrillator is available, apply and follow voice prompts.

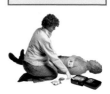

If casualty shows signs of life, turn into recovery position.

Keep checking signs of life and manage any injuries and shock until medical aid arrives.

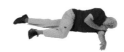

NOTE

CPR is given to a casualty when there are no signs of life – not breathing, not responding and not moving.

Compressions should be performed with the casualty on a firm surface. For an infant under one year, this is best done on a table or similar surface.

During CPR (combining chest compressions with rescue breathing), you would expect to achieve 5 sets of 30 compressions and 2 breaths (30:2) in about 2 minutes.

CPR (cardiopulmonary resuscitation)

Adult/child (over 1 year)

1   **Giving compressions:**
   - kneel beside casualty, one knee level with head and the other with casualty's chest
   - locate lower half of sternum (breastbone) in the centre of chest

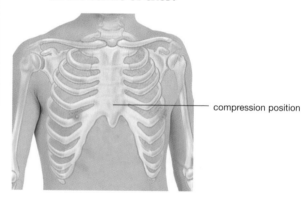

compression position

   - place heel of hand on lower half of sternum (breastbone) and place heel of other hand on top of first
   - interlock fingers of both hands and raise fingers
   - do not apply pressure over casualty's ribs, upper abdomen or bottom part of sternum
   - position yourself vertically above casualty's chest
   - with your arms straight, press down on the sternum (breastbone)
   - press down about one third of chest.

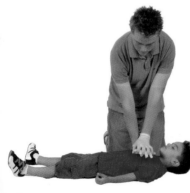

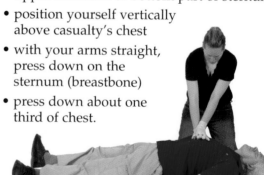

4

Infant (under 1 year)

• place two fingers (index and middle) over lower half of sternum (breastbone)

• press down about one third of chest.

2 **Release the pressure:**
• compressions and release should take equal amounts of time.

3 **Repeat compressions:**
• give 30 compressions at a rate of approximately 100 per minute.

4 **Giving breaths:**
• tilt head and lift chin (slightly for infants)
• give 2 breaths *(see p. 8).*

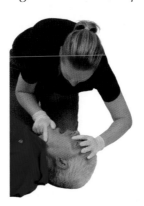
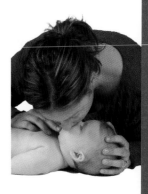

5 **Continue CPR:**
• return hands (fingers for infants) to correct position on chest
• continue compressions and breaths at a ratio of 30:2 until medical aid arrives.

5

Airway and breathing

1 **Check in mouth:**
   - if casualty is on back, leave in position
   - open mouth and look for foreign material
   - if casualty is lying face down, turn into recovery position to check for foreign material *(see p. 10)*.

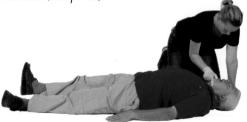

2 **If foreign material is present in the mouth:**
   - turn casualty into recovery position *(see p. 10)*
   - tilt head backwards turning slightly downwards to allow drainage of foreign material
   - clear with fingers (only remove dentures if loose or broken)

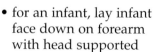

   - for an infant, lay infant face down on forearm with head supported
   - clear mouth with your little finger.

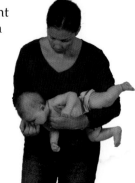

3   If mouth is clear of foreign material:
- check for breathing
- look and feel for chest movement
- listen and feel at mouth for sounds of breathing.

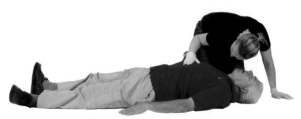

4   If casualty is breathing:
- place in recovery position *(see p. 10)*
- ☎ *call 000 for an ambulance*
- check regularly for continued signs of life until ambulance arrives.

5   If casualty is not breathing:
- ensure that ambulance has been called
- give 2 initial breaths *(see p. 8)*
- check for signs of life – breathing, response and movement.

NOTE

When giving breaths, if chest does not rise, recheck mouth and remove any obstruction. Ensure head tilt, chin lift and adequate seal around the mouth (or mouth/nose).

Giving breaths

1   Leave or place casualty onto back.

Adult/child (over 1 year)

2   Open airway:

- place your hand on the casualty's forehead, tilt head backwards

- pinch soft part of the nose closed with the index finger and thumb, or seal nose with your cheek

- open casualty's mouth and maintain chin lift

- place thumb over the chin below lip, supporting the tip of the jaw with the knuckle of middle finger

- place your index finger along jaw line

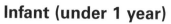

Infant (under 1 year)

- tilt head back very slightly

- lift chin to bring tongue away from back of throat

- avoid pressure under chin.

8

3   Give 2 initial breaths:
- take a breath and place your lips over the casualty's mouth (over mouth and nose for infant or small child)
- ensure a good seal
- blow steadily for about one second

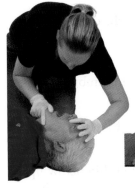 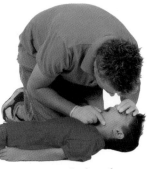 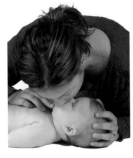

- watch for chest to rise
- maintain head tilt and chin lift
- turn your mouth away from the casualty's mouth
- watch for chest to fall
- listen and feel for signs of air being expelled.

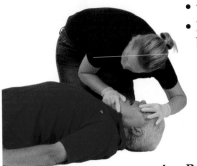 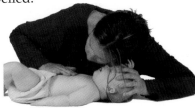

4   Repeat sequence:
- take another breath and repeat the sequence to give two breaths.

5   Check for signs of life:
- check if casualty is breathing, moving and responding
- if no signs of life, start CPR *(see p. 4)*

WARNING

If casualty has head or neck injuries, ensure head and neck is supported at all times.

DO NOT allow rotation between head and spine.

Recovery position

Adult/child (over 1 year)

1   **Position casualty's arms:**
   • kneel beside casualty
   • place farther arm at right angles to body
   • place nearer arm across chest.

2   **Position casualty's legs:**
   • lift nearer leg at knee so it is fully bent upwards.

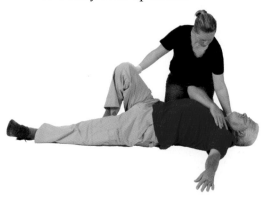

3   **Roll casualty into position:**
   • roll casualty away from you on to side while supporting head and neck.

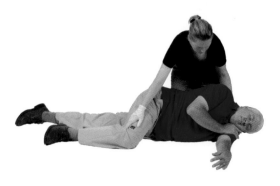

4   Prevent casualty from rolling on to face:
- keep leg at right angles with knee touching ground.

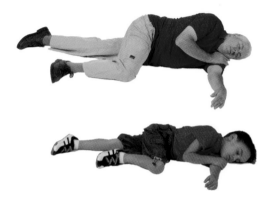

Infant (under 1 year)

- lay infant face down on an adult's forearm
- support head with hand.

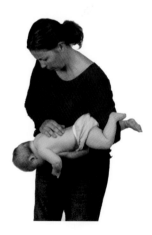

WARNING

DO NOT operate a defibrillator in a moving vehicle or in the presence of flammable substances/air mixture.

Ensure that defibrillation is performed on a non-conductive surface.

Radio frequency (RF) interference from devices such as cellular phones and two-way radios should not be used within 2 metres of an AED.

St John Ambulance conducts defibrillation training in every state and territory. Call 1300 360 455 to book into a course.

Defibrillation

There are a number of Automated External Defibrillators approved for use in Australia and while each one is slightly different, they all follow the same basic approach. Users should follow the visual and/or voice prompts of the particular AED being used.

Decide to use an AED, if the casualty:
• is unresponsive (unconscious)
• is not breathing and not moving.

If you are alone with the casualty, follow the **DRABCD** Action Plan, call 000 for an ambulance and collect the AED if available.

If two rescuers are present, one should go for help and collect the AED, if available, while the other assesses the casualty and provides Basic Life Support until the AED arrives:
• establish casualty has no signs of life
• expose the casualty's chest
• place pads on casualty's chest (follow machine's instructions)
• press 'On' button (if relevant to model of defibrillator)
• Stop CPR
• ensure everyone is clear of casualty
• follow the machine's voice prompts.

If the casualty responds to defibrillation, continue CPR until the casualty pushes the rescuer away or it is clear that there are signs of life. Do not remove defibrillator pads (even if casualty is conscious).

WARNING SIGNS

Heart Attack Warning Signs

The warning signs of heart attack vary. The symptoms usually last for at least 10 minutes. The casualty may get more than one of these symptoms:

- discomfort or pain in the centre of the chest. It may come on suddenly, or start slowly over minutes. It may be described as tightness, heaviness, fullness, or squeezing. The pain may be severe, moderate or mild

- pain may spread to the neck and throat, jaw, shoulders, the back and either or both arms.

The casualty may have other signs and symptoms including:

- shortness of breath

- sweating

- nausea/vomiting

- dizziness.

NOTE: *Cardiac arrest may occur as the first symptom of heart attack for some people – however most experience some warning signs.*

The presence of the warning signs of heart attack is a life threatening emergency.

1   **Advise casualty to rest:**
- advise casualty to stop activity, and sit or lie down and rest.

2   **Casualty to take medication:**
- if casualty has been prescribed medication such as a tablet or oral spray for angina, get it and assist the casualty in taking it as they have been directed.

3   **Seek urgent medical attention:**
- if unconscious follow DRABCD
- if symptoms last 10 minutes, get worse quickly or are severe, call 000 for an ambulance immediately
- do not drive casualty to hospital, in case of cardiac arrest.

4   **Give aspirin:**
- give 300mg (one tablet) of aspirin in water do not give aspirin to those allergic to it, to those on anti-coagulant medication (e.g. warfarin) or if their doctor has warned against them taking aspirin.

5   **Stay with the casualty and monitor vital signs:**
- monitor consciousness, breathing and movement be prepared to give CPR.

13

Common causes of choking:

- eating or drinking too quickly

- not chewing food sufficiently

- swallowing small bones

- swallowing small objects.

SIGNS & SYMPTOMS

- clutching the throat

- coughing, wheezing, gagging

- difficulty breathing, speaking or swallowing

- making a whistling or 'crowing' noise or no sound at all

- face, neck, lips, ears, fingernails turning blue

- collapsing or unconscious.

Choking

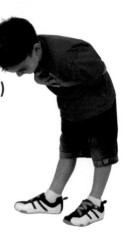

Adult/child (over 1 year)

1 **Remove object:**
   - encourage casualty to relax and breathe deeply
   - ask casualty to cough to remove object.

2 **If coughing does not remove the blockage:**
   - ☎ *call 000 for an ambulance*
   - bend casualty well forward
   - give up to 5 sharp blows with the heel of one hand in the middle of the back between shoulder blades
   - check if obstruction has been relieved after each back blow.

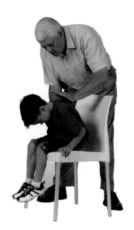

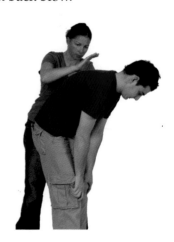

NOTE

Chest thrusts are given at the same compression point and similar to chest compressions as for CPR but sharper and delivered at a slower rate.

Chest thrusts may be given to children from one year and adults in the standing or sitting position. Infants should be placed on a firm surface on their back or held with their head low.

Continue to check the casualty until recovery or deterioration occurs. Deterioration may be recognised by the casualty becoming blue, limp or unconscious. If this occurs **call 000** and ask for an ambulance. Commence CPR.

3 **If blockage has not cleared after 5 back blows:**

- place one hand in the middle of the casualty's back for support
- place heel of the other hand in the CPR compression position on chest
- give 5 chest thrusts—slower but sharper than CPR compressions
- check if obstruction has been relieved after each chest thrust.

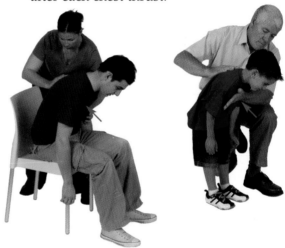

4 **If blockage has not cleared after 5 chest thrusts:**

- continue alternating five back blows with five chest thrusts until medical aid arrives.

5 **If casualty becomes unconscious:**

- remove any visible obstruction from mouth
- commence CPR

Choking

Infant (under 1 year)

1 ☎ *Call 000 for an ambulance.*

2 **Give back blows:**
- place infant with head downwards on your forearm
- support head and shoulders on your hand
- hold infant's mouth open with your fingers
- give up to 5 sharp blows between shoulders with heel of one hand
- check if obstruction has been relieved after each back blow

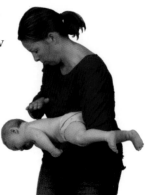

- if obstruction relieved, turn infant onto back, remove any foreign material that may have come loose with your little finger.

3   **If blockage has not cleared after
    5 back blows:**
    - place infant on back on a firm surface
    - place 2 fingers in the CPR position
    - give 5 chest thrusts—slower but sharper
      than CPR compressions
    - check if obstruction has been relieved
      after each chest thrust.

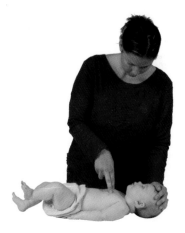

4   **If blockage has not cleared after
    5 chest thrusts:**
    - continue alternating 5 back blows with
      5 chest thrusts until medical aid arrives.

5   **If infant becomes unconscious:**
    - commence CPR.

Severe bleeding

1 **Apply pressure to the wound:**
   - remove or cut casualty's clothing to expose wound
   - apply direct pressure over wound—instruct casualty to do this if possible
   - if casualty is unable to apply pressure, apply pressure using a pad or your hands (use gloves if available)
   - squeeze the wound edges together if possible.

2 **Raise and support injured part:**
   - lie casualty down
   - raise injured part above level of heart
   - handle gently if you suspect a fracture.

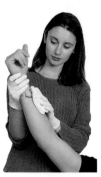

3 **Bandage wound:**
   - apply a pad over the wound if not already in place
   - secure with bandage—ensure pad remains over wound
   - if bleeding is still not controlled, leave initial pad in place and apply a second pad—secure with bandage
   - if bleeding continues, replace second pad and bandage.

4 **Check circulation below wound.**

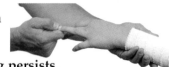

5 **If severe bleeding persists, give nothing by mouth:**
   ☎ *call 000 for an ambulance.*

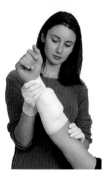

6 **Treat for shock:**
   - *(See p. 21).*

NOTE

Anaphylaxis occurs after exposure to an allergen (such as food, insect sting or medicine) to which a person is already extremely sensitive *(see p. 309)*.

SIGNS & SYMPTOMS

- swelling and redness of the skin

- itchy, raised rash (like hives)

- swelling of the throat

- wheezing and/or coughing

- rapid, irregular pulse

- tightness in the chest

- headache

- vomiting and diarrhoea

- dizziness or unconsciousness.

WARNING

An allergic reaction may be potentially life-threatening.

Allergic Reaction (Anaphylaxis)

1 Follow DRABCD.

2 If the casualty is carrying an EpiPen®, for the allergy, it should be used at once:
   - where State and Territory legislation permits, administer the EpiPen® according to the recommended Anaphylaxis Action Plan *(see website: www.allergy.org.au).*

3 ☎ *Call 000 for an ambulance.*

4 Keep casualty in lying or sitting position.

5 Observe and record pulse and breathing.

6 If conscious:
   - help casualty to sit in position that assists breathing.

   If unconscious:
   - check for signs of life and prepare to give CPR if necessary.

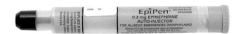

Note: Some people are aware of their hypersensitivity, so check (e.g. in a handbag) for a syringe of adrenaline (EpiPen®).

19

Asthma attack

If casualty is unconscious
- follow DRABCD
- ☎ *call 000 for an ambulance*

If casualty is conscious

1   **Make casualty comfortable:**
- help casualty into comfortable position— usually sitting upright and leaning forward
- ensure adequate fresh air
- tell casualty to take slow, deep breaths.

2   **Help with administration of casualty's medication:**
- give 4 puffs of a blue reliever inhaler— casualty takes a breath with each puff
- use a spacer if available; give 4 puffs, one at a time—casualty takes 4 breaths after each puff
- wait 4 minutes
- if no improvement, give another 4 puffs.

3   **If attack continues:**
- ☎ *call 000 for an ambulance*
- for a severe attack, until ambulance arrives, keep giving:

children   4 puffs every 4 minutes

adults   6–8 puffs every 5 minutes.

- weak, rapid pulse
- cold, clammy skin
- rapid breathing
- faintness/dizziness
- nausea
- pale face, fingernails, lips.

Shock

1 **Assess casualty:**
   - follow DRABCD, calm casualty
   - manage injuries such as bleeding.

2 ☎ *Call 000 for an ambulance.*

3 **Position casualty:**
   - raise legs over level of heart
   (unless fractured or a snake bite).

4 **Treat any other injuries:**
   - stop bleeding; treat wounds, burns,
   - immobilise fractures.

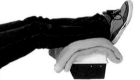

5 **Ensure comfort:**
   - loosen tight clothing around neck, chest and waist
   - maintain body warmth
   - if casualty is conscious, does not have abdominal trauma and unlikely to require an operation immediately, give small amounts of clear fluid (preferably water) frequently.

6 **Monitor and record breathing and pulse.**

7 **Place casualty in recovery position:**
   - place in recovery position if casualty has difficulty breathing, is likely to vomit or becomes unconscious *(see p. 10).*

21

Burns

1   **Remove casualty from danger:**
   - follow **DRABCD**
   - if clothing on fire:
     STOP, DROP AND ROLL
     - pull casualty to ground
     - wrap in blanket or similar
     - roll casualty along ground until flames extinguished.

2   **Cool the burnt area:**
   - hold burnt area under cold running water—up to 20 minutes
   - if a chemical burn, run cold water over burnt area—at least 20 minutes
   - if a bitumen burn, run cold water over burnt area for 30 minutes
   - if burn is to eye, flush eye with water for 20 minutes.

3   **Remove any constrictions:**
   - remove clothing and jewellery from burnt area (unless sticking to the burn).

4   **Cover burn:**
   - place sterile, non-stick dressing over burn.

5   **Calm casualty.**

6   ☎ *Call 000 for an ambulance.*

Snake and spider bite

Snake/funnel-web/mouse spider

1   **Check breathing and circulation:**
- if casualty unconscious, follow **DRABCD**.

2   **Calm casualty.**

3   **Apply pressure immobilisation bandage:**
- apply a firm roller bandage starting just above the fingers or toes and moving up the limb as far as can be reached
- bandage needs to be very firm.

4   **Immobilise casualty:**
- apply a splint to immobilise bitten limb
- check circulation in fingers or toes
- ensure casualty does not move.

5   ☎ *Call 000 for an ambulance.*

Red-back spider

1   **Apply icepack to bitten area and seek medical aid.**

SIGNS & SYMPTOMS

- abdominal pain
- drowsiness
- nausea/vomiting
- burning pains from mouth to stomach
- difficulty in breathing
- tight chest
- blurred vision
- odours on breath
- change of skin colour with blueness around lips
- sudden collapse.

WARNING

DO NOT attempt to induce vomiting.

Cyanide poisoning
If breathing stops, wash mouth and lips Commence **CPR**. (**DO NOT** inhale casualty's expired air)

Poisoning

If casualty unconscious:
1   Follow DRABCD.

2   ☎ *Call 000 for an ambulance.*

3   Call fire brigade if atmosphere contaminated with smoke or gas.

If casualty conscious:
1   Check for danger.

2   Listen to casualty:
- give reassurance but not advice.

3   Determine nature of poisoning.
- try to determine type of poison take, and record.

4   ☎ *Call 000 for an ambulance.*

5   Call 13 11 26 for Poisons Information Centre.

SIGNS & SYMPTOMS

- altered or abnormal responses to commands and touch

- wounds to the scalp or face

- blood or clear fluid escaping from nose or ears

- pupils becoming unequal in size

- blurred vision

- loss of memory.

WARNING

Wear gloves, if possible, to protect against infection.

If bleeding does not stop, without disturbing dressing, reposition pad and reapply pressure to control bleeding.

Head injury

1 **Monitor breathing and pulse:**
- if casualty unconscious, follow **DRABCD**
- keep casualty's airway open with fingers (if face badly injured).

2 **Support head and neck:**
- support casualty's head and neck during movement in case the spine is injured.

3 **Control bleeding:**
- place sterile pad or dressing over wound
- apply direct pressure to wound unless you suspect a skull fracture
- if blood or fluid comes from ear, secure a sterile dressing lightly in place and allow to drain.

4 **Lie casualty down:**
- place casualty in comfortable position with head and shoulders slightly raised
- be prepared to turn casualty onto side if they vomit
- clear the airway quickly after vomiting.

5 ☎ *Call 000 for an ambulance.*

SIGNS & SYMPTOMS

- pain at or below site of injury

- loss of sensation, or abnormal sensation such as tingling, in hands or feet

- loss of movement or impaired movement below site of injury.

WARNING

If casualty unconscious, place in recovery position.

If casualty conscious, do not move, but support head.

Spinal injury

1   **Swift immobilisation is highest priority:**
   - do not move casualty unless in danger.

2   **Check breathing and circulation:**
   - if casualty unconscious, follow **DRABCD**.

3   **Support casualty's head and neck at all times:**
   - place hands on side of head until other support arranged

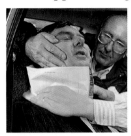

   - apply a cervical or improvised collar to minimise neck movement.

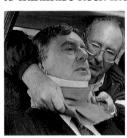 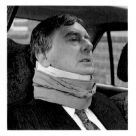

4   **Give reassurance:**
   - calm casualty.

5   ☎ *Call 000 for an ambulance.*

Eye injury

1   **Support casualty's head:**
   - support casualty's head to keep it as still as possible
   - ask casualty to try not to move eyes.

2   **Flush eye with cool, flowing water:**
   - if chemical or heat burn, or smoke in eyes, flush with water.

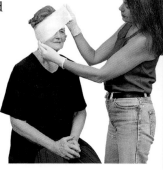

3   **Place dressing over eye:**
   - place a sterile pad or dressing over injured eye
   - ask casualty to hold this in place
   - bandage dressing in place, covering injured eye
   - if a penetrating eye injury, lie casualty on back, place pad around object and bandage in place.

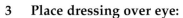

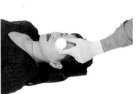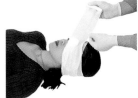

4   ☎ *Call 000 for an ambulance.*

SIGNS & SYMPTOMS

Fracture and dislocation

- pain at or near the site of the injury

- difficult or impossible normal movement

- loss of power

- deformity or abnormal mobility

- tenderness

- swelling

- discolouration and bruising.

Fractures, dislocations, sprains and strains

FRACTURES AND DISLOCATIONS

1   Follow DRABCD.

2   Control any bleeding and cover any wounds.

3   Check for fractures:
    - open, closed or complicated.

4   Ask casualty not to move injured part.

5   Immobilise fracture:
    - use broad bandages (where possible) to prevent movement at joints above and below the fracture
    - support the limb, carefully passing bandages under the natural hollows of the body
    - place a padded splint along the injured limb (under leg for fractured kneecap)

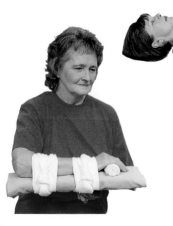

    - place padding between the splint and the natural contours of the body and secure tightly
    - check that bandages are not too tight (or too loose) every 15 minutes.

NOTE

If collarbone is fractured, support arm on injured side in a St John sling.

If dislocation of a joint is suspected, rest, elevate and apply ice to joint.

It can be difficult for a first aider to tell whether the injury is a fracture, dislocation, sprain or strain. If in doubt, always treat as a fracture.

6   For leg fracture, immobilise foot and ankle:
     • use figure of eight bandage.

7   Watch for signs of loss of circulation to foot or hand.

8   ☎ *Call 000 for an ambulance.*

SPRAINS AND STRAINS

1   Follow DRABCD.

2   Follow RICE management plan:
     R — rest
     I — ice
     C — compression
     E — elevation.

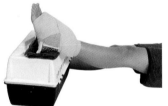 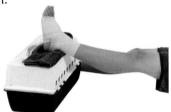

3   Seek medical aid.

29

SIGNS & SYMPTOMS

- feeling hot, exhausted and weak

- persistent headache

- thirst and nausea

- giddiness and faintness

- fatigue

- rapid breathing and shortness of breath

- pale, cool, clammy skin

- rapid, weak pulse.

Additional symptoms

- high body temperature

- flushed skin

- irritability and mental confusion may progress to seizure and unconsciousness.

WARNING

Heatstroke may develop.

Heat-induced conditions

Heat Exhaustion

1   Lie casualty down:
- move casualty to lie down in a cool place with circulating air.

2   Loosen tight clothing:
- remove unnecessary garments.

3   Sponge with cold water.

4   Give fluids to drink.

5   Seek medical aid:
- if casualty vomits
- if casualty does not recover promptly.

Heat Stroke

1   Follow DRABCD.

2   Apply cold packs or ice:
- apply to neck, groin and armpits.

3   Cover with wet sheet.

4   ☎ *Call 000 for an ambulance.*

5   If casualty is fully conscious and is able to swallow, give fluids.

Hypothermia

1 Follow DRABCD.

2 Remove casualty to a warm, dry place.

3 Protect casualty:
- protect casualty and yourself from wind, rain, sleet, cold, and wet ground.

4 Avoid excessive activity or movement.

5 Maintain casualty in horizontal position.

6 Remove wet clothing.

7 Warm casualty:
- place between blankets or in sleeping bag, and wrap in space blanket or similar.

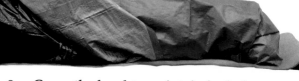

8 Cover the head to maintain body heat.

9 Give warm drinks if conscious:
- do not give alcohol.

- fever

- twitching of face or limbs

- eyes rolling up

- congestion of face and neck

- blue face and lips

- stiffness of body with arched back

- unconsciousness.

WARNING

DO NOT cool child by sponging or bathing.

Infantile convulsions

1 **During convulsions:**
- place child on floor for safety
- turn child on side
- do not restrain child.

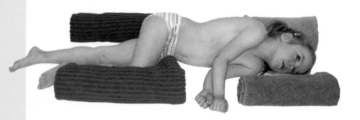

2 **After convulsions:**
- follow **DRABCD**
- remove excess clothing or wrapping
- seek medical aid.

SIGNS & SYMPTOMS

Low blood sugar

- pale
- hungry
- sweating
- weak
- confused
- aggressive.

High blood sugar

- thirsty
- needs to urinate
- hot dry skin
- smell of acetone on breath.

Diabetic emergency

If casualty unconscious:

- follow **DRABCD**
- ☎ *call 000 for an ambulance.*

If casualty conscious, and signs suggest low blood sugar:

- give sweet food or drink (not diet, diabetic or sugar-free drinks) every 15 minutes until casualty recovers or medical aid arrives
- ☎ *call 000 for an ambulance.*

If casualty conscious, and signs suggest high blood sugar:

- allow casualty to self-administer insulin—do not administer it for them but assist if required
- ☎ *call 000 for an ambulance*
- give casualty sugar-free fluids to drink, if help delayed.

NOTE: If you are not sure which form of diabetic emergency the casualty has, give a sweet drink. If casualty has a high blood sugar emergency, then giving a sweet drink will not do undue harm.

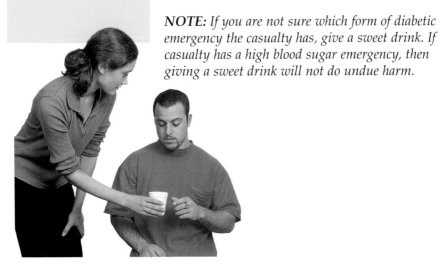

Epileptic seizure

1   **Check breathing and circulation:**
- follow **DRABCD**.

2   **Protect casualty:**
- protect from injury
- do not restrict movement
- do not place anything in mouth.

3   **Manage injuries:**
- place on side as soon as possible
- manage injuries resulting from seizure
- do not disturb if casualty falls asleep
- continue to check for signs of life.

4   **Seek medical aid if:**
- the seizure continues for more than 5 minutes
- another seizure quickly follows
- the person has been injured.

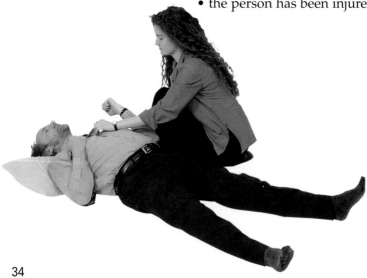

2

The emergency situation

2

What is first aid?

First aid skills are based on knowledge, training and experience. First aid is the initial care of the ill or injured and usually is given by someone who is on the spot when a person becomes ill or injured. The skills of first aid are for all.

At any time, you may find yourself in a situation where someone has had an accident or is suffering from a sudden illness and needs help until a qualified health care professional such as a doctor, registered nurse or ambulance paramedic arrives.

The aims of first aid are to:
- promote a safe environment
- preserve life
- prevent injury or illness from becoming worse
- help promote recovery
- provide comfort to the ill or injured.

A first aider should:
- assess the situation quickly
- identify the nature of the injury or illness as far as possible
- arrange for emergency services to attend
- manage the casualty promptly and appropriately
- stay with the casualty until able to hand over to a health care professional
- give further help if necessary.

Nature of the injury or illness

Sometimes the nature of the injury or illness, unpleasant smells, or the sight of blood, vomit, or torn skin may be distressing. This is natural; even ambulance paramedics and doctors sometimes experience these reactions.

To prepare yourself, take a few deep breaths and look away from the injuries prior to administering first aid. Act confidentley—the skills you provide will help to save this person's life.

Medical aid

Medical aid is the treatment by a health care professional—doctor, registered nurse or ambulance paramedic. Medical aid takes over from first aid when the health professional arrives at the scene of an incident. The first aider may be required to remain and assist if requested by the health care professional.

Other first aiders

The first aider who arrives first at the scene of an incident takes charge and stays in charge until handing over control. Any other first aider who arrives should offer to help the original first aider, without trying to take control. If you feel another first aider at the scene is more qualified to handle the situation, ask that person to take control. However, the most qualified person does not need to be in control, especially if another first aider already has matters well in hand.

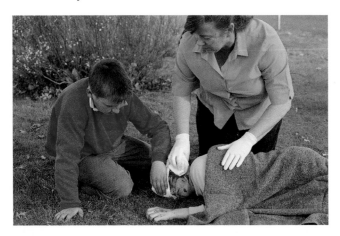

The casualty

You may feel uncertain about touching someone who is a stranger, who is of a different age group, race, or sex, or is from your workplace. Your ability to deal with the emergency and perhaps save the person's life will depend on your ability to put aside these concerns and deal with the emergency in the best way you can.

A casualty's behaviour may also cause you to be hesitant about giving first aid. The casualty may be acting strangely or be uncooperative. Sometimes a casualty may act in an offensive manner as a result of the injury or illness, or because of stress or the influence of alcohol or other drugs. Attempt to establish a rapport with the casualty by introducing yourself and asking the casualty's name. If the casualty's behaviour prevents you from giving help, there are still things you can do:

- Make sure someone has called the appropriate emergency services.
- Try to reassure and calm the casualty.

If at any time the casualty's behaviour poses a threat to you, withdraw from the scene. If necessary, monitor from a safe distance and make sure other bystanders are safe.

Consent to first aid treatment

Before you provide any first aid to a casualty, you must first gain the consent from the casualty to begin the treatment. If the casualty is unresponsive and therefore unable to give consent, it is presumed that they would have given the consent if they were conscious. If the casualty is a child, the parent/guardian should be asked for permission, but if the parent/guardian is not present and the injury/illness is life-threatening, immediate first aid should be given. A written record of the first aid management should be kept.

Duty of care

When you have made the decision to give first aid and have commenced first aid treatment on a casualty, you have committed yourself to provide a duty of care to that casualty. This duty of care requires that you remain and provide first aid treatment to the casualty to the best of your ability and to your level of training until another or more experienced first aider takes over, medical aid arrives or you are physically unable to continue to provide first aid to the casualty or the situation becomes unsafe to do so.

Infection control

The actual risk of disease transmission in first aid is extremely low. Nevertheless, you should take some simple steps to protect both yourself and the casualty from the risk of infection. By using standard precautions such as wearing disposable gloves to prevent direct contact with bodily fluids while giving first aid, and by washing your hands thoroughly before, if possible, and straight after giving first aid even if you have been wearing gloves, you are observing 'best practice' health care. If you do come into contact with a casualty's bodily fluids, seek medical advice as soon as possible. Chapter 6 provides some further information on infection control.

Smoking in relation to first aid

At a first aid scene, St John Ambulance Australia discourages smoking by first aiders, casualties and bystanders because of the possible presence of flammable fuel and the use of medical gases.

Managing an accident scene

In an emergency, your involvement as a trained first aider may be crucial. Sometimes bystanders are reluctant to act at an emergency because they may be unsure of what to do. Therefore, it is very important that time is not lost in getting emergency care to the casualty and administering the necessary first aid. The calm, controlled manner of a confident first aider will ensure that the management of the scene is handled effectively and efficiently and that:

- casualties are protected from further injury
- first aiders and caregivers are protected from injury
- there is easy access for emergency services
- efficient treatment and evacuation of casualties to hospital occurs
- priorities for casualty management are assessed.

If the site is well managed, more lives can be saved. As a trained first aider, it may be more effective for you to manage the entire situation rather than help only one person.

Emergencies attract the attention of a lot of people who may stand around and watch. To give the casualty the safest care possible, only those people really needed should be at the scene. These include:

- any witnesses to the incident
- relatives and close friends of the casualty
- any bystanders you ask to stay to help.

Everyone else should be asked to move well away. Always look for bystanders who can help in some way. A bystander may be able to:

- help make the scene safe
- call 000 for the emergency service(s) required for the incident and/or local authorities (e.g. to have power turned off)
- give you information on the casualty's medical problems or allergies
- gain information from the casualty, bystanders and anyone else who can help
- find a first aid kit or alternative materials
- gather and protect the casualty's belongings
- ease concerns of the casualty's relatives and friends
- calm, reassure and help protect the privacy of the casualty
- provide necessary information to emergency personnel
- warn traffic to slow down or stop if trained to do so
- help give first aid
- secure the area from onlookers.

Notification of an emergency incident

Any traffic accident or other emergency incident should be reported to the emergency services as soon as possible. Call 000 for an ambulance and police and any other service required. If there is a damaged powerline, advise the emergency services call taker to ensure that the electricity authority is also contacted.

Emergency number—Call 000

It is important to be able to give emergency services all the information they require about the location of the accident, number of casualties and types of injuries. Consider the following:

- Which emergency service do you need?
- Always ask for an ambulance first, then police.
- Who else is needed at the accident site?
- How many people are involved?
- Advise if anybody is trapped.
- Is there a danger from high-voltage wires?
  - ask for electricity authority to be contacted.
- Is there a danger from chemical or fuel spillage, a gas leak or fire?
  - ask for fire services.

It is important that the following information is provided about the location of the accident:

In a city or town, provide:
- street number
- street name
- landmarks (e.g. cross street)
- suburb
- city/town
- state/territory.

In a rural area, provide:
- distance from intersection/landmark/roadside number
- road
- area
- nearest city/town
- landmark
- state/territory.

2

Information required by emergency services

When calling emergency services:
- make sure you have all the necessary information before speaking to the operator
- keep messages brief and accurate
- ensure messages are not given too quickly, are clear and can be easily understood
- be the last to hang up.

Calling emergency services

1 **Call 000** for an ambulance. If using a mobile phone and 000 does not work, try 112.

2 Ask for the ambulance service (ambulance will call other services if required).

3 Give the exact place of the accident with directions.

4 Give the approximate number of casualties.

5 Give an indication of the type and extent of injuries where possible.

6 State if any other emergency services are required.

7 Give the telephone number of the phone you are using.

8 Ask the likely time of arrival of the ambulance service.

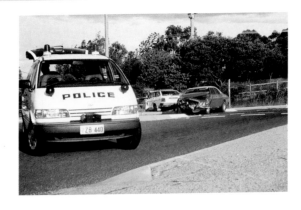

Accidents where first aid is required

There are many accident settings requiring first aid. The most common first aid scenario is a traffic accident. The following actions apply for all types of accidents. At a traffic accident involving two to three casualties, the first aider will need to assess each casualty's injuries and situation (e.g. whether trapped in a vehicle) to determine an order of priority for first aid management. Your decisions about where casualties with serious injuries are most likely to be located and the injured casualties that will most likely need urgent attention may literally be a matter of life or death. Such decisions frequently need to be made on the basis of limited information and in situations of critical urgency.

Airway management has the highest priority. If a casualty is found to be unconscious while seated in a car at the scene of an accident, simply lifting the chin and moving the jaw forward will open the casualty's airway and allow them to breathe.

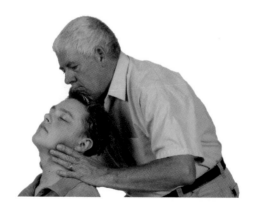

A major traffic accident may involve multiple types of small and large vehicles. First aid management may be limited by resources available at an accident scene, particularly when there are multiple casualties, or if the arrival of emergency services is delayed. In rural areas, people involved in a traffic accident are at greater risk; hence the importance of calling emergency services as soon as possible. It is important to prioritise casualties according to the degree of urgency for the purpose of first aid management and evacuation (this is called triage). The aim is for the most good to be done for the largest number of people and only applies to a situation where there are more casualties than the first aider can manage. Chapter 24 provides comprehensive information about how to triage and manage accidents involving multiple casualties.

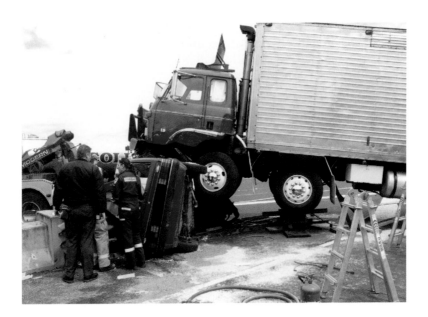

Safety at the scene

The emergency scene must be made safe for everyone—
yourself, bystanders and the casualty.

You will need to determine if:

- there is any continuing danger (e.g. fallen powerlines)
- anyone's life is in immediate danger (e.g. from a fire or
  flammable materials).

Leave dangerous situations for emergency personnel to deal
with as they have the training and equipment to do so.
However, after assessing the situation, remove the danger
or prevent new dangers whenever possible. For example, if
a child has received an electric shock at home, turn off the
electricity immediately at the power point or at the main
switchboard. At the scene of a road traffic accident, authorities
will need to remove the power source.

At the scene of a road traffic accident, you can position other
cars with their hazard lights flashing to warn oncoming traffic
of the danger. At night it is also recommended that headlights
are switched on to illuminate the scene. If at any time you
suspect the scene is unsafe, it is better to wait for emergency
personnel to arrive and ensure all bystanders are clear of the
scene rather than place yourself and others in danger.

At an accident, distraught or potentially violent people may
be experiencing an emotional reaction to the accident, or
to a loved one seriously injured, trapped in the vehicle,
or even dead. These people need special consideration at a
major accident scene. They have to be cared for, and perhaps
prevented from interfering with the management and removal
of other casualties. If people at the accident scene are physically
uninjured, but very agitated, or preventing the first aider from
attending to serious injuries, they need to be removed gently
but firmly. A suitable bystander can be recruited to escort
them away from the accident scene and to try to calm and
reassure them.

2

Assessing the danger

At an accident site, first aiders must make an assessment
of the possible danger to themselves and to any casualties.

Dangers to look for include:
- other traffic
- fire
- fumes
- damaged vehicles
- spilt fuel or chemicals
- fallen or damaged high-voltage overhead powerlines
- unstable structures (e.g. powerlines or buildings).

Other traffic

Other traffic is always of primary concern. The accident
site has to be protected so that no further accidents occur.
To warn other vehicles:
- safely park a car at a suitable distance from accident
- put on hazard lights
- if at night, use headlights to illuminate the scene
- if there is a bystander at the scene who is trained to control
  traffic, ask them to warn and control oncoming vehicles.

Fire

Fire can start in any badly damaged vehicle, particularly if
electrical wiring is damaged or fuel spilt. To prevent fires:
- switch off the vehicle's ignition
- shut off the emergency fuel switch of a diesel vehicle
- prevent anyone smoking near the accident site.

Obtain a fire extinguisher, if possible, and have it ready. If there
is a fire under the bonnet of a vehicle, release the bonnet catch
(if possible), but do not open the bonnet fully. Aim the fire
extinguisher through the gap towards the flames.

Fumes

Fumes from leaking petrol can cause an explosion. Bystanders should be kept well away and no naked flames or smoking allowed.

Damaged vehicle

A damaged vehicle can be dangerous. The following precautions should be taken:

- Stay clear of the steering wheel and front dashboard of a vehicle fitted with airbags if those airbags have not been activated.
- Put on handbrake.
- Put vehicle in gear (if not already).
- Place blocks against wheels.

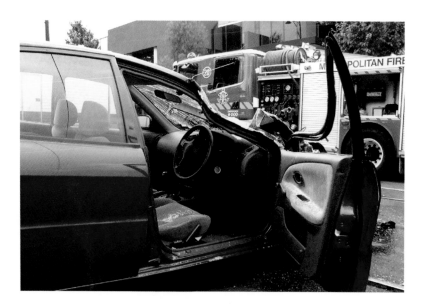

2

Spilt fuel or chemicals

Where an accident involves a vehicle carrying hazardous materials, the rule is to stay clear of the accident scene. However, emergency services must be notified and care taken by the first aider to secure the safety of the scene. Without putting yourself in danger, note:

- clouds of vapour
- spilt liquids, bottles, gas cylinders
- unusual odours.

Vehicles containing hazardous substances will have display notices or signs indicating the contents. When notifying emergency services, give:

- code number (HAZCHEM Emergency Action Code)
- type of sign.

Avoid contact with these substances and stay upwind to avoid breathing in any toxic fumes.

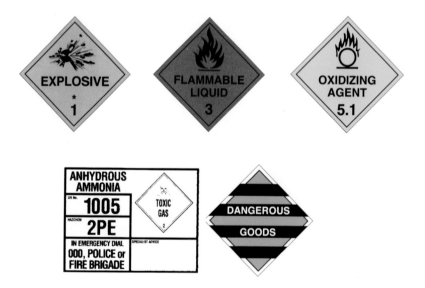

2

Fallen or damaged high-voltage overhead powerlines

High-voltage electricity can be a serious hazard at an accident site. If a car has hit a light or electricity pole, high-voltage powerlines can be knocked down and may even come into contact with the vehicle. If this has happened:

- remain at least 6 metres from any cable (high-voltage electricity can arc up to 6 metres)
- ensure bystanders do not go within 6 metres of cable
- call emergency services
- DO NOT attempt to move cable
- DO NOT go near a vehicle or try to remove a person from a vehicle being touched by a high-voltage cable. Advise the casualty not to move. Wait for emergency services to arrive.

There is considerable risk that, if a fallen cable is touching a vehicle, it could catch fire. If it becomes necessary, due to fire or other external life-threatening situation for anyone in the vehicle, to get out, they should do so only if they can jump clear without touching the vehicle and the ground at the same time. Otherwise, they will act as an earth for the electricity and may be killed.

In most situations, anyone inside the vehicle should be told to remain there until the danger from the electrical cable has been removed.

Other cars can be used to warn oncoming vehicles that there is an accident ahead. Cars not involved in the accident or not being used to warn oncoming traffic should be cleared from the site if possible. Phones, two-way radios and CB radios are often available in cars, taxis, interstate transports, and courier vehicles. These can be used to contact emergency services.

Types of injuries

The injuries you are likely to have to deal with will vary according to the type of accident. The most common form of care required is simple comfort and reassurance. An airway blockage often occurs with those involved in an accident as casualties may be thrown forward by the force of the impact. Other injuries may include head and chest injuries for adults and injuries to the head for children.

Pedestrians often have multiple injuries. Head and spinal injuries are common and often fatal. If run over, the pedestrian may have a crushed chest, abdomen or pelvis. There may also be injuries from being dragged under a car.

Bicyclists have a high risk of head injury, especially if not wearing a helmet. They often have severe arm and leg injuries and sustain injuries similar to pedestrians when hit by a vehicle.

Motorcyclists are the most likely of all road users to suffer a spinal injury resulting in paralysis. They may also have large areas of skin stripped off by the road or other hard surface. These injuries are particularly prone to infection because they contain a lot of embedded dirt and debris.

Priorities of casualty management

In dealing with an accident, illness or any other situation that requires the help of a first aider, it is important to determine which injuries or conditions are most in need of your attention. In the primary assessment, determine whether the casualty:

- is conscious (moving around) or unconscious
- airway is clear and open
- is breathing
- is bleeding.

Unconsciousness is a life-threatening condition

If the casualty is unconscious:

- the airway may be blocked if the tongue has relaxed and fallen to the back of the throat (causing breathing to stop and, soon after, the heart to stop beating)
- there is risk of choking as the casualty has no ability to swallow or cough out any object
- the capacity for self-protection from potential dangers (e.g. traffic, fire, a collapsing building, drowning) may be lost.

When there is more than one casualty, you will have to assess quickly which casualty takes priority. This will mean assessing which are the most serious injuries and which of these need immediate attention. A noisy, demanding casualty may be a lower priority than the silent casualty who may have a blocked airway.

The decisions you make about which casualty most urgently needs help may be influenced by factors not related to their injuries. If one of the seriously injured casualties is trapped in a car, it may be difficult for you to give more than minimal first aid. In such a situation, you may decide that someone else who is not as seriously injured has priority.

Movement of a casualty

Unless absolutely necessary do not move a casualty until medical aid arrives. Moving a casualty unnecessarily may lead to further injury. If the casualty's life is endangered (e.g. by the risk of an explosion, drowning, or collapse of a burning building), remove the casualty from the scene by the quickest and safest means available, regardless of injuries or the manner in which removal must be made. If a neck or spinal injury is suspected, support for the neck must be provided before moving *(see p. 259).*

Before you act, consider:
- the dangerous conditions at the scene
- the casualty's size
- your own health and physical ability
- if there are others who can help
- the casualty's condition.

This will help you decide the best method to use for moving the casualty, whether you need assistance and whether other aids such as a blanket are needed.

When injuries appear to be serious or extensive, seek medical aid urgently. Road or air ambulance is the preferred method of transporting the seriously injured casualty. Improvised transport may endanger the casualty's chance of survival and should only be used if no ambulance is available.

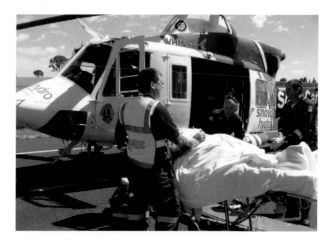

Removal of helmets

A traffic accident may involve someone who is wearing a motorcycle helmet or other type of protective headgear. A full-face helmet should be removed only if absolutely necessary i.e. if you are unable to maintain the casualty's airway or if resuscitation is required. Half-face helmets and full-face helmets with a chin piece that lifts up should be left on with the chin strap either cut or removed to ensure a clear airway.

Management of helmet removal

Note: Removal of helmets should be performed by two people.

1 Place the casualty on their side, supporting head and neck to avoid any twisting during movement.

5 Carefully and gently continue to tilt the helmet backwards and forwards until the helmet is off the casualty's head.

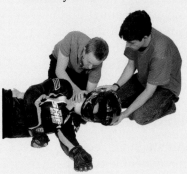

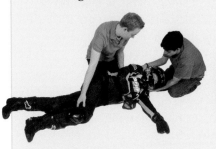

2 Unfasten or cut the helmet chin strap.

3 Carefully and gently tilt the helmet back to pass over the chin.

6 Be careful not to catch the helmet on the casualty's ears or nose.

7 Place the helmet next to the casualty so that it can be given to the ambulance personnel.

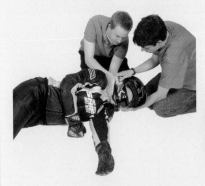

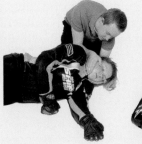

4 Carefully and gently tilt the helmet forward to pass over the back of the head.

2

After the emergency

In first aid we prepare ourselves for all types of emergency situations, but we don't always think about what happens after the casualty has left our care. Once you have handed the casualty over to the ambulance or a doctor, there may be a number of practical things that need attention. These may include cleaning up the accident scene, and correcting any unsafe conditions that caused the accident. This is usually performed by emergency services personnel. If you are a workplace first aid officer and the incident is workplace related, you may be required to write a report.

Post-traumatic stress

Although life seems to go back to normal following an incident, many people think back over a stressful event and try to evaluate what more they could have done. The more serious the incident, the more you are likely to think about it. This is completely normal. However, if it continues for weeks or begins to affect your day-to-day life, you may be experiencing post-traumatic stress.

Post-traumatic stress is a possible reaction to a stressful event. It needs to be dealt with, as it can affect your relationships, your concentration and your peace of mind. You should consult your doctor or a counsellor. They will understand what you are going through and will be able to suggest a course of action to help you deal with the effects of post-traumatic stress.

General principles of casualty management

Emergencies often result in confusion. Those nearby may not know what to do first, who should take charge or how to get help. The following sequence of actions will help ensure that safe and appropriate first aid is given.

1   Initial assessment based on the **DRABCD** Action Plan.

2   Calling for medical assistance.

3   History from the casualty.

4   Secondary casualty assessment.

5   Ongoing casualty care.

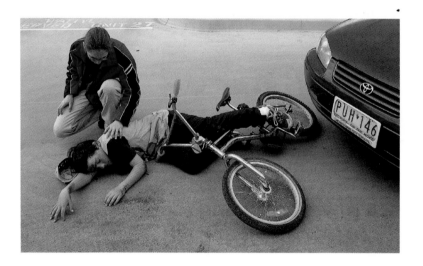

2

DRABCD Action Plan

The St John **DRABCD** Action Plan is a vital aid to the first aider in casualty management.

D - **Danger**
R - **Response**
A - **Airway**
B - **Breathing**
C - **CPR**
D - **Defibrillation**

This plan helps you find out:
- what dangers are present to you, bystanders and the casualty
- how many casualties are involved
- what immediate first aid is required
- what caused the injury
- if the casualty is conscious or unconscious
- if the airway is clear and open
- if the casualty if breathing
- if resuscitation is needed.

The detailed implementation of **DRABCD** is set out in chapter 3, Basic Life Support.

Once you have applied the principles of **DRABCD**, and if necessary phoned for an ambulance or sent someone to call for help, proceed to gain a history of events leading up to and of the incident from the casualty and complete a secondary assessment.

History from the casualty

When you are taking a history from a casualty, the aim is to find out anything that may be important about the casualty and the situation:

- **events leading to incident**—ask how the incident happened
- **symptoms**—find out casualty's symptoms such as pain and nausea
- **allergies**—ask if casualty has any allergies
- **past medical history**—check for a Medic Alert® bracelet or anything that could relate to the current injury or illness
- **medication**—ask if casualty has taken any medication in the last 24 hours or takes regular medication and if they are carrying it
- **last meal**—ask when casualty last had anything to eat or drink.

2

Secondary assessment

A secondary assessment involves carrying out a head-to-toe examination of the casualty to determine what injuries are present and prioritise the first aid treatment required according to the severity of injuries. The first aider should be especially sensitive to the age, gender and race of the person being examined.

1   Examine head
    • check for blood, bruising and swelling
2   Check face
    • check eyes (compare size of pupils, look for bruising, cuts and swelling)
    • compare one side of face to the other
3   Check neck
    • check for injuries—bruising, cuts
    • check collarbones—breakages, bruising
4   Check shoulders, arms and hands
    • check for wounds, bleeding and fractures
    • check shoulder joints and shoulderblades
    • check full length of each arm
    • check hands and each finger for bruising, swelling, cuts, breaks and feeling
5   Check chest
    • check for injuries—bruising, cuts
    • does chest expand easily and evenly?
    • does breathing cause pain?

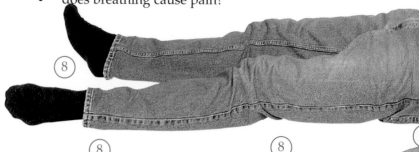

6 Check abdomen
- check for injuries—bruising, cuts
- is it tender—does a gentle press on the abdomen cause pain?

7 Check pelvis and buttocks
- check for injuries—bruising, cuts
- push tops of hips towards each other—does this cause pain?
- check for evidence of wet pants or blood from genital area

8 Check legs, ankles and feet
- check right along each leg for bruising, swelling, cuts, breaks, and abnormal alignment
  - check foot and each toe for bruising, swelling, cuts, breaks and feeling

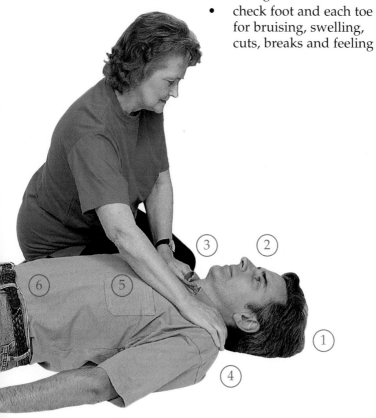

2

Ongoing assessment and care of the casualty

In any emergency there is the possibility that a casualty will be unconscious or partially conscious (often referred to as an 'altered conscious state').

If a person is unconscious or partially conscious, this indicates that something serious and possibly life-threatening is wrong. The brain is the controlling organ of the body and regulates all body functions. Any injury serious enough to alter the consciousness of the casualty may have caused damage to the brain. Unconsciousness or an altered conscious state can be caused by:

- direct injury to or illness affecting the brain as a result of:
  - head injury
  - a stroke
  - fits/seizures
  - meningitis
- lack of oxygen to the brain as a result of:
  - not breathing
  - irregular heartbeat
  - blood loss
  - severe respiratory problems including asthma
  - a blocked airway
  - allergic reaction (anaphylaxis)
  - smoke inhalation
- poisons and toxic products in the blood as a result of:
  - diabetes
  - kidney and/or liver failure
  - overdose of alcohol or other drug.

Usually the loss or partial loss of consciousness is temporary. However, a casualty may be left permanently brain damaged by any of these conditions. Good assessment and management of an unconscious or partially conscious casualty can not only save life but can also make all the difference to the future quality of life for survivors.

The principles for managing an unconscious casualty are the same as for a conscious casualty. Conscious casualties need constant reassurance and explanation of what is happening. Until medical aid arrives, the level of consciousness must be assessed as frequently as possible and recorded.

Principles of managing a casualty

The general management of casualties is the same, whatever the cause. The casualty needs:

- protection from danger
- to be in a recovery position (for unconscious casualties)
- a clear airway
- injuries treated such as bleeding, burns or wounds
- medical aid—**call 000** for an ambulance
- signs of life (response, breathing and movement) monitored until ambulance arrives.

In addition to monitoring signs of life until medical aid is available, it is useful to also record the casualty's observations including breathing, pulse, skin colour and temperature. A record of the casualty's observations will assist with their ongoing care. Any change in the casualty's observations could indicate a serious change in their condition.

Breathing observation

Normal respiration is quiet, regular, and effortless and may be slower and shallower during sleep. Observations made of breathing include the rate, rhythm and character. The rate is the number of times the casualty breathes in and out. The rhythm is the regularity of respirations (breathing in and out at regular intervals). The character is the way a person breathes. Depending on the casualty's condition, this may include slow, rapid, shallow or wheezing respirations.

Breathing is counted by observing the rise and fall of the casualty's chest (one count for each rise and fall) and noting the rhythm and character. Try to count breaths without the casualty being aware.

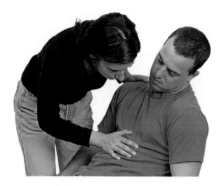

Pulse observation

The pulse is the beat of the heart felt through the distension of an artery wall. The rate, rhythm and volume of the pulse is observed. The rate is the number of heartbeats felt. The rhythm is the regularity of the heartbeat. Some irregularities may be observed as a missed beat, double beats then a long pause or a quivering pulse. The volume is the strength of the heartbeat. A normal pulse should be strong enough so it is not easily compressed. Abnormalities may include a full, bounding or a weak, thready pulse.

The pulse may be observed at the neck (carotid), groin, wrist (radial) or inner upper arm of an infant (brachial pulse). The pulse is most often taken at the wrist by placing the index and middle fingers over the inner side of wrist at the base of the thumb and applying enough pressure to feel the heartbeat. The pulse is counted for one minute while observing the rhythm and volume at the same time.

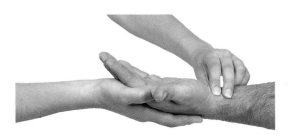

Skin colour and temperature observation

A casualty's skin colour and temperature can suggest a variety of medical conditions. Some conditions may cause the skin colour to be red, white, blue or yellow and may be clammy or wet. It is important to record the initial observation of skin colour and condition and if or when changes occur. Observing the skin temperature may be achieved by feeling with the back of your hand if a digital thermometer is not available.

Checklist for managing an unconscious casualty

Ensure area is clear of danger

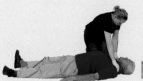 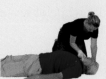 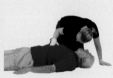 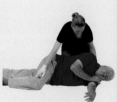

Check for response
No response

Check in mouth
Mouth/airway
is clear

Check breathing
Breathing is present

Recovery position
Support head
and neck
Open airway

Manage life-threatening injuries:
external bleeding, burns, wounds

Send for
medical aid
(if possible do not
leave an unconscious
casualty alone)

Monitor signs of life:
response, breathing and movement

Carry out a head-to-toe examination

Take and record observations:
breathing, pulse, temperature
and skin colour

Manage other injuries

Ask bystanders
what happened

Check pockets, wallet or purse for
ID, medication, Medic Alert®
bracelet or necklet etc.

Record all
observations

3

Basic life support

Basic life support is essentially the ABC of emergency care. It is the action taken to maintain airway, breathing and circulation, and thereby life itself, in the hope that the natural function of the lungs and heart will be restored. If there are no signs of life, cardiopulmonary resuscitation (CPR) must be quickly applied or the casualty is certain to die.

There are three main actions in providing basic life support:

1   Maintain an airway—this may involve having to clear an obstruction, such as the tongue, foreign material or vomit from the airway.

2   Give two initial breaths to inflate a casualty's lungs by breathing into casualty's mouth.

3   Give external cardiac compressions carried out in a rhythmical fashion combined with breaths.

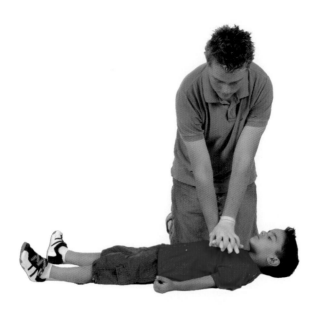

These simple techniques will either restart normal heart action or maintain circulation sufficient to preserve brain function until specialised assessment and treatment are available. If the casualty is unconscious and breathing, ensuring the airway is open takes precedence over any other injury. However, it is important to handle the casualty gently with a minimum of movement.

If you are faced with an emergency in which there is a life-threatening situation, what you do in the first few minutes will be critical. It is important that the call for the ambulance is performed as soon as possible in an emergency. If the casualty is an infant or small child, take them with you to make the call.

Direct contact with the casualty's mouth during rescue breathing, especially if vomit or blood is present, can be avoided with the use of personal protection items such as a pocket mask (see p. 87) or a face shield. However, rescue breaths should not be delayed by attempts to obtain personal protection equipment.

Basic life support is the preservation or restoration of life by the establishment and maintenance of the airway, breathing and circulation. It is closely linked to the chain of survival providing immediate actions following a cardiac arrest. The time taken to call for help and provide basic life support skills—CPR and AED—is vital.

Chain of survival

Immediate action needs to be taken to maximise a casualty's chances of survival, particularly when there are no signs of life. This 'chain of survival' is the key to improving the survival rate from cardiac arrest in our community. Time is of the essence!

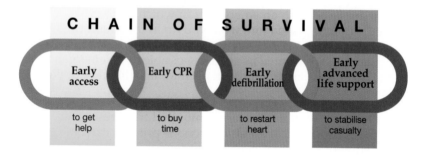

What is the chain of survival?

Early access
The ambulance must be called immediately to ensure that early defibrillation and advanced life support can commence without delay.

Early CPR
If CPR is begun within 4 minutes of the heart stopping, oxygenation of the vital organs (such as the brain) is maintained.

Early defibrillation
If CPR is given within 4 minutes and defibrillation within 8–12 minutes, there is a significantly improved chance of survival.

Early advanced life support
Definitive treatment by the ambulance service, such as giving medication and stabilising the airway, may increase chances of survival even further.

The DRABCD Action Plan

The St John **DRABCD** Action Plan is a vital aid to the first aider in assessing whether the casualty has any life-threatening conditions and if any immediate first aid is necessary.

D   check for **DANGER**
- to you
- to others
- to casualty

R   check **RESPONSE**
- is casualty conscious?
- is casualty unconscious?

A   check **AIRWAY**
- is airway clear of objects?
- is airway open?

B   check for **BREATHING**
- is chest rising and falling?
- can you hear or feel air from mouth or nose?
- if not breathing, give 2 initial breaths

C   give **CPR**
- if no signs of life—unconscious, not breathing and not moving, give CPR
- CPR involves giving 30 compressions at a rate of approximately 100 compressions per minute followed by 2 breaths.

D   apply a **DEFIBRILLATOR** (if available)
- follow voice prompts

D DANGER

In every emergency situation, it is important to see if there are any conditions that may be an immediate threat to life. It is most important to make sure the area is safe for yourself, others and the casualty. Dangers such as obstacles, electrical wires, gas or toxic fumes can cause serious injury; a flue leak from a stove or heater can cause the carbon monoxide level in a room to become dangerously high. Make sure that you do not become a casualty too—you are no help to the casualty if you become injured yourself. Once you have made sure the area is safe, you can go ahead with assessing the casualty.

R RESPONSE (consciousness)

The next step is to determine if the casualty is conscious:

1   Ask casualty for their name.

2   Gently squeeze casualty's shoulders.

OR

Ask casualty to squeeze
your hands (both
sides should be tried
if a stroke is suspected).

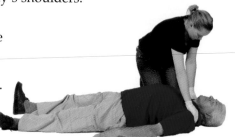

A response indicates that the casualty is conscious and can be left in the position in which you found them (provided there is no further danger).

1   Manage any life-threatening injuries that need
    immediate attention.

2   Manage other injuries.

3   Get help if injuries require it.

4   Calm the casualty.

No response indicates that the casualty is unconscious and it is important to get help as quickly as possible as unconsciousness is a life-threatening condition.

If another person is available, ask them to **call 000** for an ambulance.

A AIRWAY

Check mouth for obstruction

It is essential to the casualty's chance of survival to ensure that the airway is clear so that breathing is possible.

An obstruction of the airway may be caused by:
- the back of tongue
- solid or semi-solid material such as food, vomit or blood
- swelling or injury of the airway.

If the casualty is lying on the back, open mouth and look for foreign material.

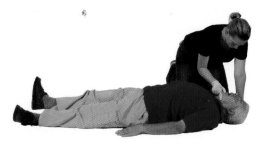

Note: *If the casualty is lying face down, turn into recovery position to check for foreign material.*

If foreign material is present in the mouth, turn the casualty into the recovery position while supporting the neck and spine.

Note: *The recovery position for an infant under 1 year of age is different from that for an adult/child (see p. 73).*

Clearing the airway

With adult/child in the recovery position—open airway gently:

1   Tilt head backwards.

2   Turn mouth slightly downwards to allow drainage of foreign material.

3   Clear foreign material with your fingers, if required. Only remove dentures if they are loose or broken.

With infant in the recovery position, clear mouth of foreign material with little finger.

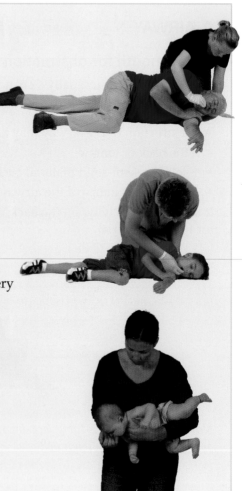

Recovery position

1 Kneel beside casualty.

2 Place farther arm at right angle to body.

3 Place nearer arm across chest.

4 Lift nearer leg at knee so it is fully bent upwards.

6 Keep leg at right angle with knee touching ground to prevent casualty rolling onto face.

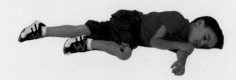

For an infant, the most suitable recovery position is lying face down on an adult's forearm with the head supported by the hand.

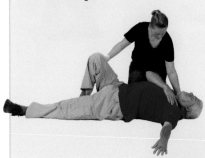

5 Roll casualty away from you onto side while supporting head and neck.

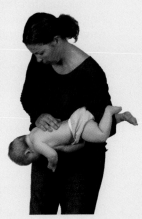

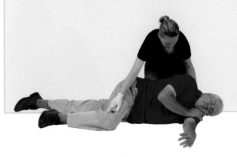

Opening the airway

With the casualty in the
recovery position if you need
to clear the mouth
of foreign material,

OR

with the casualty on their back
if the airway is clear:

Adult/child (over 1 year)

1　Place your hand high on
the casualty's forehead.

2　Place thumb of your other
hand over chin below lip,
supporting the tip of jaw
with knuckle of middle
finger. Place your index
finger along jaw line.

3　Gently tilt the head
backwards to bring tongue
away from back of throat.

4　Lift the chin, opening the
casualty's mouth slightly.

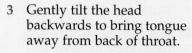

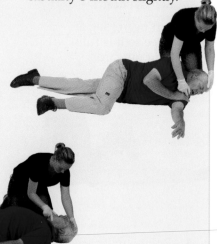

Infant (under 1 year)

1　Place infant flat on back.

2　Tilt head back very slightly
to open the airway.

3　Lift chin to bring tongue
away from back of throat.

4　Avoid pressure on
soft tissue under
infant's chin.

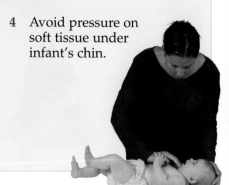

If a casualty is found to be unconscious in a seated position (e.g. car accident or slumped in chair), simply lifting the chin and moving the jaw forward will open the casualty's airway allowing them to breathe.

B BREATHING

Check for breathing:

1   Look and feel for chest movement.
2   Listen and feel for sounds of air escaping from the mouth and nose (an occasional gasp is not adequate for normal breathing).

Note: Take no more than 10 seconds to do this.

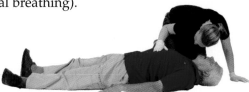

If the casualty is breathing:

•   place casualty in recovery position *(see p. 73)*

•   **call 000** for an ambulance

•   check regularly for continued signs of life until medical aid arrives.

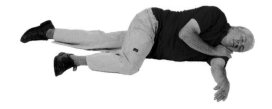

If the casualty is NOT breathing:

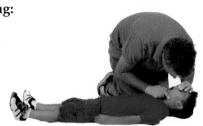

- ensure the call to 000 for an ambulance has been made

- give 2 initial breaths

- check for signs of life.

Note: *If you are alone, place casualty in a recovery position with airway open—call 000 for an ambulance.*

C CARDIOPULMONARY RESUSCITATION (CPR)

Cardiopulmonary resuscitation is the technique of compressions of the chest (pushing down on the lower half of the casualty's breastbone) and inflation of the lungs (breathing into the casualty's mouth). CPR is given to a casualty when there are no signs of life—not breathing, not responding and not moving.

If the casualty shows signs of life, but is unconscious:

- turn onto side into the recovery position
- continually check the casualty's condition until medical aid arrives (call for help if not already done)
- be ready to turn casualty onto back and start CPR if breathing stops.

If there are no signs of life commence CPR.

1   Give 30 compressions *(see p. 81)*.

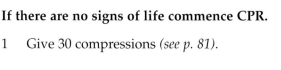
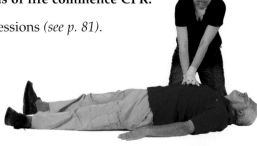

2   After 30 chest compressions,
    tilt head and lift chin.

3   Give 2 breaths *(see p. 79)*.

4   Return your hands (fingers
    for infants) immediately to
    correct position on sternum.

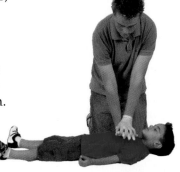

5   Give a further 30 compressions.

6   Continue compressions and
    breaths in a ratio of 30:2 until
    medical aid arrives.

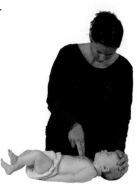

*Note: If a first aider is unwilling or unable to perform
rescue breathing, compression-only CPR will be better
than not doing CPR at all.*

Change over between first aiders during CPR

When two first aiders are present or if a second
person arrives to help:

- ensure that an ambulance has been called
- one of the two first aiders indicates readiness or
  a need to change
- the first aider must change over smoothly with minimal
  interference to the resuscitation procedure
- change should be done frequently, approximately every
  two minutes, to minimise fatigue.

When to stop CPR

You can stop giving CPR when:

- the casualty shows signs of life
- more qualified help arrives
- you are physically unable to continue.

When the casualty shows signs of life

1   Turn the casualty to the recovery position.

2   Call for ambulance or medical aid as soon as possible
    (if not done already).

3   Assess casualty for bleeding and other injuries noting
    tenderness, swelling, wounds or deformity in the
    following order:
    - head, face and neck
    - shoulders, arms and hands
    - chest
    - abdomen
    - pelvis and buttocks
    - legs, ankles and feet.

4   Continue monitoring for **DRABCD**.

Rescue breaths

The air you breathe out of your lungs contains about 16% oxygen. This amount of oxygen breathed into the casualty's lungs, combined with compressions during CPR will preserve the circulation of air and blood around the body while waiting for medical aid to arrive.

Giving rescue breaths

1   Leave or place casualty onto back.

2   Open airway.

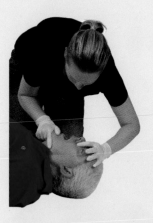

Adult/child (over 1 year)

-   Place your hand on the casualty's forehead, tilt head backwards and pinch soft part of the nose closed with the index finger and thumb, or seal nose with your cheek.

-   Open the casualty's mouth and maintain chin lift— place thumb over the chin below the lip, supporting the tip of jaw with the knuckle of middle finger. Place your index finger along jaw line.

Infant (under 1 year)

-   Tilt head back very slightly and lift chin to bring tongue away from back of throat avoiding pressure under chin.

3 Take a breath and place your lips over the casualty's mouth, ensuring a good seal. If a small child or infant, place your lips over mouth and nose. Blow steadily for about one second.

4 Watch for chest to rise.

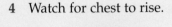
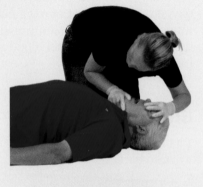
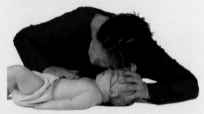
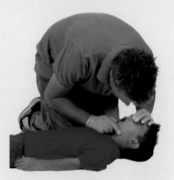
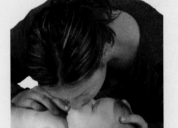

5 Maintain head tilt and chin lift.

6 Turn your mouth away from the casualty's mouth—watch for chest to fall, and listen and feel for signs of air being expelled.

7 Take another breath and repeat the sequence.

Note: *If the chest does not rise, recheck the mouth and remove any obstructions, ensure adequate head tilt and chin lift and ensure there is an adequate seal around the mouth (or mouth/nose).*

Giving compressions

Compressions should be performed with the casualty on a firm surface. In the case of an infant this is best done on a table or similar surface.

1 Adult/child—kneel beside casualty, one knee level with head and the other with casualty's chest.

2 Locate lower half of sternum (breastbone) in the centre of chest.

Adult/child (over 1 year)

- Place heel of hand on lower half of sternum (breastbone) and place heel of other hand on top of first.

- Interlock fingers of both hands and raise fingers to ensure that pressure is not applied over casualty's ribs, upper abdomen or bottom part of sternum.

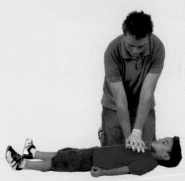

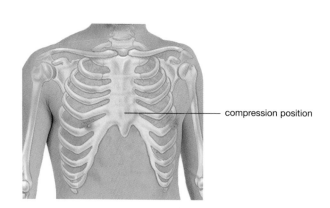

compression position

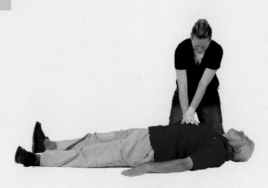

3 Position yourself vertically above casualty's chest.

4 With your arms straight, press down on the sternum (breastbone) to depress about one third of chest.

5 Release the pressure (compressions and release should take equal amounts of time).

6 Repeat to complete 30 compressions at a rate of approximately 100 per minute.

Infant (under 1 year)

- Place two fingers (index and middle) over lower half of sternum (breastbone).

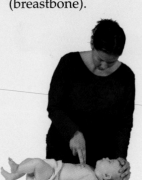

Note: *During CPR (combining chest compressions with rescue breathing), you would expect to achieve 5 sets of 30 compressions and 2 breaths (30:2) in about 2 minutes.*

D DEFIBRILLATION

The second D of the St John Action Plan emphasises
the importance of attaching a defibrillator if available.
A defibrillator is used to treat sudden cardiac arrest, a
condition that occurs when the heart stops pumping. Use
of a defibrillator is the third link in the chain of survival.
This indicates that it is vital that the cardiac arrest casualty is
defibrillated as quickly as possible. Many situations requiring
cardiopulmonary resuscitation (CPR) are due to the heart
fibrillating. A defibrillator can detect this and will give an
electric shock if required. This may restore normal heart rhythm.

CPR can maintain the blood flow and keep the blood
oxygenated. Sudden cardiac arrest is usually caused by
fibrillation, a disturbance of the electrical activity in the heart's
ventricular muscle, or larger pumping chamber. This causes the
heart to quiver or 'fibrillate' in a disordered way. The electrical
disruption prevents the heart pumping blood around the body
effectively causing the heart to stop beating, leading to a
cardiac arrest. With the use of a defibrillator, an electric shock
can be delivered to restore the heart's electrical activity. It is
crucial that CPR continues at all times, except when the actual
electric shock is being delivered.

Following successful defibrillation, CPR should be continued
until the casualty pushes the rescuer away or it is clear that
there are signs of life.

Note: *St John Ambulance conducts defibrillation training in every
state and territory. Call 1300 360 455 to book into a course.*

Drowning

A person gasping for air while trying to stay afloat may inhale only a small amount of water. The casualty usually has little water in the lungs because the muscles of the larynx (voice box) close the airway to stop water entering. However, the spasm which prevents water going in also prevents air from going in. Mucous plugs form. As a result, the casualty suffocates and becomes unconscious. Every second is vital in management of drowning.

Infants and children can drown very quickly if they are left unattended in a bath, near a swimming pool, pond or spa, or the beach, near a river, canal or dam. There is a better than fifty per cent chance of saving an apparently drowned infant or child by giving CPR.

It is important to remember that even in the case of a successful rescue, qualified personnel should be called as the casualty will still need to be assessed and monitored.

Note: If you encounter a person drowning and if you do not have the swimming abilities or strength to effect the rescue, use 'non-contact' rescue techniques e.g. shout, reach out, throw a float, wade out and try to reach the casualty.

Casualty in a wheelchair

If the casualty is in a wheelchair and requires CPR, carefully and safely take the casualty out of the wheelchair and place onto back to commence CPR. Consideration needs to be given to the possible fragile nature of the casualty's bones, and use of correct manual handling techniques by the first aider to prevent back strain.

Pregnant casualty

If a woman requiring CPR appears to be in an advanced state of pregnancy:

- position her on her back with shoulders flat

- place padding under her right buttock to tilt pelvis to the left

- if there is not enough padding available to achieve a definite tilt, a second person should hold the casualty's abdomen to the left side while CPR is performed.

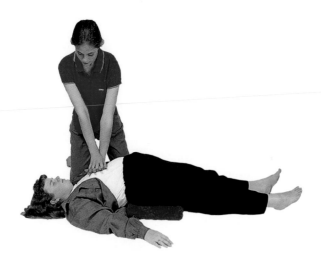

Other methods for giving breaths

Mouth-to-nose breaths

The mouth-to-nose technique is used when:
- the jaw and/or teeth are broken
- the jaws are tightly clenched
- resuscitating in deep water
- resuscitating an infant or small child when your mouth can cover the casualty's nose and mouth together.

1   Kneel beside the casualty.

2   Keep the casualty's head tilted back.

3   Close the casualty's mouth.

4   Place your thumb on the lower lip to keep the casualty's mouth closed.

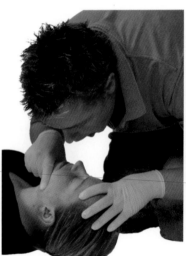

5   Support the jaw.

6   Take a deep breath and open your mouth wide.

7   Seal your mouth around the casualty's nose (infant—mouth and nose) without compressing the soft part.

8   Blow into the casualty's nose (infant—mouth and nose).

9   Remove your mouth and allow the casualty's mouth to open by removing your thumb to allow exhalation.

Mouth-to-mask breaths

The mouth-to-mask technique, using a resuscitation mask, avoids mouth-to-mouth contact between the first aider and the casualty. This is especially appropriate if the casualty has vomited, if blood is present or if the casualty is inebriated. However, resuscitation should not be delayed by attempts to obtain a mask.

1   Kneel beside the casualty, one knee level
    with head and the other with casualty's chest.

2   Tilt head backward, lift chin and support jaw
    to maintain an open airway.

3   Place narrow end of mask on bridge of nose
    (apply mask firmly to achieve an effective seal).

4   Take a deep breath and blow through the mouthpiece
    of the mask.

5   Remove your mouth to allow exhalation.

6   Turn your head to listen and feel for the
    escape of air.

7   If the chest does not
    rise, recheck head tilt,
    jaw support and
    mask seal.

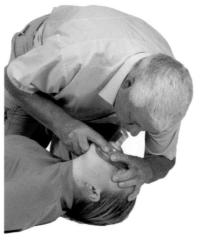

Mouth-to-stoma

Mouth-to-stoma breaths are performed on casualties who breathe totally through the stoma (neck breathers) or partially through a stoma, mouth and nose (partial neck breathers). A stoma is a hole in the windpipe visible in the front of the neck resulting from a partial or total removal of the larynx (voice box). This procedure is usually done as part of the treatment for cancer, but sometimes after burns, injury or infection.

A cravat, scarf or other fabric filter over the neck may alert the rescuer to the possible presence of a stoma. A stoma will be more obvious when the casualty is on the back. If a tube is seen in the stoma, always leave it in place to keep the hole open for breathing and resuscitation.

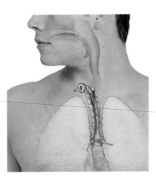

total neck breather

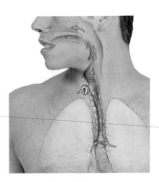

partial neck breather

1   Support the jaw with the head in backward tilt to make it easier for you to seal your mouth over the stoma.

Note: For a partial neck breather, seal the nostrils with index and middle fingers and use the thumb to press the chin upwards and backwards, sealing the lips.

2   Take a deep breath and blow through the stoma—watch for rise and fall of chest.

Note: For a partial neck breather—when the chest rises, lift the fingers sealing the nose and mouth and listen for escaping air from nostrils and stoma.

If the chest fails to rise, this may be due to:

- a poor seal over the stoma
- air is escaping from mouth and nose from a partial neck breather
- stoma or tube is blocked—do not remove the blocked tube. If foreign material is obvious, attempt to clear it. Reattempt inflation by blowing harder. If still blocked, use back blows and chest thrust in an attempt to dislodge the obstruction *(see p. 92).*

DANGER

Check for Danger – ensure scene is safe

RESPONSE

Check for Response

| RESPONSE

Make comfortable Monitor signs of life | NO RESPONSE
Open mouth—look for foreign material |

AIRWAY

| NO FOREIGN MATERIAL
Leave on back
Open airway | FOREIGN MATERIAL
Recovery position
Open and clear airway |

BREATHING

Check for Breathing

| BREATHING
Place in recovery position. Call **000** for an ambulance
Monitor signs of life | NOT BREATHING
*Call 000** for an ambulance

Give 2 initial breaths
Check for signs of life |

CPR

| SIGNS OF LIFE
Recovery position
Monitor signs of life | NO SIGNS OF LIFE
Start CPR—
30 compressions and 2 breaths |

DEFIBRILLATION

Apply AED
Give 1 shock
Repeat CPR for about 2 minutes
Follow voice prompts

Note: If you are alone and casualty is not breathing, place in recovery position before calling 000.

CPR = Cardiopulmonary Resuscitation
AED = Automated External Defibrillator

Choking (airway obstruction)

A person chokes when the airway is partly or completely blocked. The casualty usually has trouble breathing and, if obstruction is complete, cannot breathe at all. Some choking casualties clutch their throat with their hands with impending suffocation. Unless given first aid, the casualty may die. The first aider's aim is to dislodge the object stuck in the throat, to clear the casualty's airway.

The most common causes of choking are:

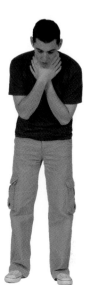

- eating or drinking too quickly
- not chewing food sufficiently
- swallowing small bones
- swallowing small objects.

Note: Many adult casualties who experience choking are also under the influence of alcohol.

SIGNS AND SYMPTOMS:

- clutching the throat
- coughing, wheezing, gagging
- having difficulty breathing, speaking or swallowing
- trying to cry but making strange sounds or no sound at all
- making a whistling or 'crowing' noise
- face, neck, lips, ears, fingernails turning blue
- turning blue in the face
- collapsing or being unconscious.

Infants and small children love to put things in their mouths. This can result in choking. Toys, food, pen caps and coins may be responsible. Peanuts and hard sweets are especially dangerous for children under five.

The simplest way to assess the severity of an airway obstruction is to check whether a cough is effective or ineffective. The casualty with an effective cough should be encouraged to keep coughing to expel the foreign material. The first aider should continue to check the casualty until recovery or deterioration occurs. Deterioration may be recognised by the casualty becoming blue, limp or unconscious. If this occurs **call 000** and ask for an ambulance—start CPR.

If the cough is ineffective, manage the casualty for choking.

Management of choking

1 Encourage adult or child (over 1 year) casualty to relax and breathe deeply.

2 Ask casualty to cough—to remove object.

If coughing does not remove the blockage, or if casualty is an infant:

1 **Call 000** for an ambulance.

2 Give 5 back blows— checking if obstruction is relieved after each back blow.

3 If unsuccessful, give 5 chest thrusts—checking if obstruction is relieved after each chest thrust.

4 If blockage does not clear after 5 chest thrusts, continue alternating 5 back blows with 5 chest thrusts until medical aid arrives.

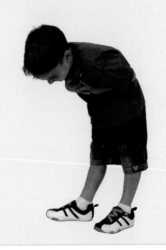

If casualty becomes unconscious:

1 **Call 000** for an ambulance.

2 Remove any visible obstruction from the mouth.

3 Commence CPR.

Giving back blows

Adult/child (over 1 year)

1 Bend casualty well forward.

2 Give up to 5 sharp blows with the heel of one hand in the middle of the back between the shoulder blades.

3 Check after each back blow to see if the airway obstruction has been relieved.

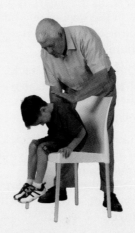

4 If blockage has not cleared after 5 back blows—give chest thrusts.

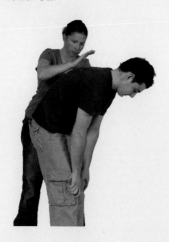

Infant (under 1 year)

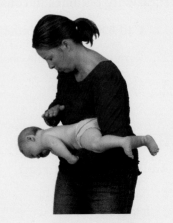

1   Place infant with head downwards on your forearm—supporting head and shoulders on your hand. Hold infant's mouth open with your fingers.

2   Give up to 5 sharp blows with the heel of one hand to the back between shoulders.

3   Check after each back blow to see if the airway obstruction has been relieved.

4   Turn infant onto back, open infant's mouth and remove any foreign material that may have come loose with your little finger.

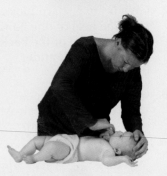

5   If blockage has not cleared after 5 back blows—give chest thrusts.

Chest thrusts

To perform chest thrusts identify the same compression point as for CPR and give 5 chest thrusts. Chest thrusts are similar to chest compressions but sharper and delivered at a slower rate. Chest thrusts may be given to children (1–8 years) and adults in the standing or sitting position. Infants should be placed on a firm surface on their back or held with their head low. If the obstruction is not relieved after 5 chest thrusts, continue alternating 5 back blows with 5 chest thrusts until medical aid arrives.

Giving chest thrusts

Adult/child (over 1 year)

1   Give 5 chest thrusts. Place one hand in the middle of the casualty's back for support and heel of other hand in the CPR compression position and give 5 chest thrusts— slower but sharper than CPR compressions.

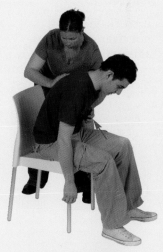

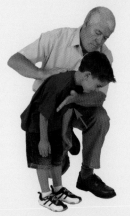

Infant (under 1 year)

1   Place on back on a firm surface. Place two fingers in the CPR compression position and give 5 chest thrusts—slower but sharper than CPR compressions.

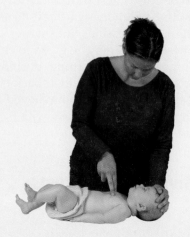

2   Check after each chest thrust to see if the airway obstruction has been relieved.

3   If blockage is still not cleared, continue alternating 5 back blows with 5 chest thrusts until medical aid arrives.

Note: If casualty becomes unconscious commence CPR.

4

Advanced resuscitation

This chapter contains information and techniques for administering extra supplemental oxygen to a casualty suffering from a medical condition or injury, resuscitation with the aid of oxygen and techniques to defibrillate a casualty following a sudden cardiac arrest.

Administration of oxygen is beneficial in the management of sick or injured casualties. Training must be undertaken to ensure there is an understanding of the regulations that govern the safe storage and use of oxygen.

Automated external defibrillators (AEDs) are becoming increasingly available in workplaces and the public domain. AEDs are used in an attempt to re-start the heart in the case of sudden cardiac arrest.

Use of oxygen in first aid

Oxygen should be given to all people suffering from a lack of oxygen (hypoxia) due to an injury, or medical condition. It is used to assist in the resuscitation of a non-breathing casualty and as therapy for a breathing casualty (e.g. someone with smoke inhalation, or asthma). Conditions for which a casualty may require oxygen include:

- unconsciousness
- shock
- head injuries
- heart attack and heart conditions
- severe injury of any type
- heatstroke
- respiratory distress
- poisoning
- gas, smoke or capsicum spray inhalation

- chest conditions (casualty not able to breathe deeply enough, and thus at risk of hypoxia)
- abdominal injuries
- eye injuries (deterioration can occur very rapidly without oxygen)
- fractures
- all other injuries—helps to reduce the extent of tissue damage as a result of insufficient oxygen.

Note: If equipment is not immediately available, start CPR without oxygen.

Oxygen cylinders

Identification

Medical oxygen cylinders are normally identified as black metal cylinders with white shoulders and clearly labelled as medical oxygen.

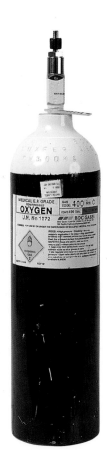

Storage of oxygen cylinders

Oxygen cylinders may be stored upright or on the side in a cool, dry ventilated area below 45° C. Ensure that cylinders are secured using appropriate brackets.

When the cylinder is almost empty (1/4 or less full), close valve, remove from oxygen equipment, mark cylinder as 'empty' or 'MT' and store away from full cylinders.

4

Care with oxygen

DO NOT drop, drag, roll or slide cylinders (if fractured, the pressure released will turn cylinder into a high-powered missile).

DO NOT use oxygen near artificial heat sources.

DO NOT allow smoking near oxygen equipment.

DO NOT use oxygen if there is any danger of fire.

DO NOT direct oxygen output towards the area of defibrillation; or have oxygen equipment switched off.

Use of oxygen cylinders

Only use a cylinder with an Australian Standards approved regulating device.

Always use correct pressure gauges with oxygen.

Ensure valve seat and seal inserts are clean, dry and in good condition.

DO NOT allow petroleum-based grease or oil to come in contact with supply devices on the stem of the cylinder.

Note: There is a high risk of combustion when oxygen is used in conjunction with oil or grease. Consequently, oil or grease MUST NOT be used on oxygen equipment.

Selecting and 'cracking' an oxygen cylinder

1   Select an appropriate size medical oxygen cylinder to suit apparatus to be used. Only medical oxygen, which is filtered and purified when cylinder is filled, should be used. Medical oxygen cylinders are normally black with white around the cylinder's neck or shoulder.

2   Select a full cylinder, ensuring that a plastic dust seal is in place over the oxygen outlet hole. Leave seal in place until oxygen cylinder is required.

The plastic seal, which usually also covers the indexing pin holes, enables the first aider to readily distinguish full cylinders from used ones. Make sure the plastic seal is intact and has not been moved.

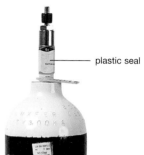

plastic seal

The most commonly used oxygen cylinders are:

- C size cylinders =   400 to 490 litres of useable oxygen
- D size cylinders =   1640 litres of useable oxygen
- Special cylinders =   approximately 200 litres of useable oxygen.

'Portable' oxygen resuscitators commonly use the C size cylinder.

Smaller cylinders such as C size cylinders have two indexing holes on the cylinder stem, for correct location of the cylinder on to the regulator which is called a pin index. These index holes prevent non-medical oxygen regulators from being used by mistake. Engage the cylinder on to the two protruding pins on the regulator's inlet face. There should be a seal between the cylinder's outlet hole and the regulator's oxygen inlet. This seal is the first location to check if any oxygen leaks are present. Listen for leaks once the cylinder clamp screw has been firmly tightened and the cylinder is turned on.

3 Before 'cracking' (opening) a cylinder, manually remove dust seal completely from full cylinder.

4 To 'crack' a cylinder:

- place the oxygen keywheel/ spanner on to keyway at end of oxygen cylinder

- explain to bystanders and casualties that you are about to crack the cylinder to avoid frightening them

- place one hand halfway down cylinder for stability; with other hand, turn oxygen outlet hole away from yourself and anyone else present—the oxygen jet can cause a nasty friction burn

- turn the keywheel slowly and gently anticlockwise until oxygen flow is heard, then quickly back to the off position, to clear dust or other contaminants from valve area.

  The new oxygen cylinder is now ready to be connected to equipment.

5 Select appropriate oxygen connecting apparatus.

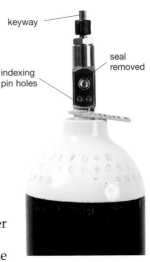

keyway

seal removed

indexing pin holes

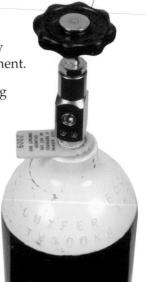

keywheel

Oxygen equipment

Assembling oxygen equipment

To permit the oxygen contained within an oxygen cylinder to be given to a casualty, the following basic components are required:

- oxygen cylinder—preferably full; usually replace for refilling when contents are 1/4 or less
- oxygen regulator—reduces oxygen cylinder pressure to a working level
- flow rate control—permits either fixed or variable flow rates of oxygen
- tubing and mask—for effective administration of oxygen to the casualty.

Before using any oxygen equipment (including masks, airway and suction equipment), it should be checked for faults and defects in accordance with the manufacturer's instructions, industry standards and regulatory requirements.

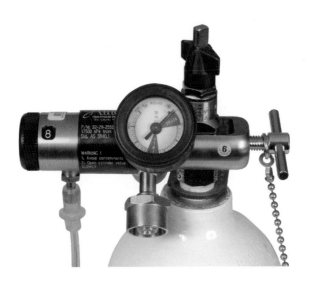

Restoring and maintaining equipment ready for future use

Whenever oxygen equipment has been used:

- precautions must be taken to ensure there is no potential for spread of infection from one casualty to another or to first aider
- prepare it again for immediate use—check regularly; turn cylinder on and off again to check contents
- discarded appropriately—oxygen equipment consumables marked for single use, such as oxygen masks, after use.

After use, clean and prepare the equipment for reuse by:

- replacing disposable components
- cleaning and sterilise non-disposable components.

After equipment has been dismantled:

- wipe regulator carefully with damp cloth
- check that the seal between the regulator housing and cylinder yoke is always correctly positioned and in good condition.

Servicing equipment

Oxygen regulators and flow valves require annual servicing. The manufacturer's recommendations for servicing should be followed.

Administration of oxygen

There is a variety of oxygen equipment available to assist spontaneously breathing casualties and provide oxygen to non-breathing casualties. It is important that you are familiar with their general characteristics. Whatever device is used, it is always important to explain to the casualty what it is and why it is necessary.

Breathing casualty

Oxygen may be administered to provide supplemental oxygen to a conscious or unconscious breathing casualty via:

- a face mask or nasal cannula with a selected and controlled oxygen flow rate
- a soft bag mask system with a reservoir bag attached and connected to an oxygen cylinder

  or

- an oxygen-powered resuscitator; demand valve system which automatically supplies 100% of oxygen as the casualty breaths in may be operated by those trained in its use.

Non-breathing casualty

Oxygen may be given to a non-breathing casualty via:

- an oxygen-powered resuscitator; demand valve system with a manual override button for inflating the lungs,

  or

- a hand-powered, soft bag mask system with a reservoir bag attached and connected to an oxygen cylinder.

Soft bag mask systems may also be operated without connecting to an oxygen cylinder in non-breathing casualties.

Infection control

Standard precautions are work practices required for basic levels of infection control. They include good hygiene practices, particularly washing and drying hands before and after casualty contact; the use of protective barriers which may include gloves, gowns, aprons, masks, eye goggles; appropriate handling and disposal of sharps and other contaminated or infectious waste; and use of aseptic techniques. If the first aider has a respiratory tract infection, or the casualty is not breathing, a face mask should be worn while treating the casualty.

Disposable protective gloves should be worn at all times to reduce the risk of exposure to blood or other likely body substances. Any exposed cuts or grazes should be covered with a waterproof or film dressing before putting on protective gloves. After use, the gloves must be taken off without touching the outside surface and, where possible, hands should be washed and dried immediately.

When oxygen administration is being given and there is more than one casualty, a new mask for each casualty is used to ensure that neither the first aider nor the casualties are placed at risk of cross-infection.

Breathing casualty

Oxygen therapy must be administered at an appropriate flow rate for the wellbeing of a casualty. To ensure this, it is important to continue to monitor the casualty throughout the procedure.

Simple universal plastic face mask (therapy)

The simple universal plastic face mask can deliver up to 60% oxygen depending on the flow rate and the speed and depth of the casualty's breathing. Exhaled air is vented through the holes on each side of the mask. At low oxygen flow rates and deep respirations the casualty may draw in room air through the side holes thereby diluting the oxygen concentrations received. As a general guide a flow rate between 8 and 15 litres per minute (lpm) should ensure adequate oxygen delivery to the casualty. A flow rate under 8 lpm with quick respirations, may not be enough to 'flush' out the carbon dioxide in the face mask fully and therefore may have an effect on respiratory effort.

Some casualties may find it difficult to tolerate a face mask and complain of suffocation when placed over the face and mouth. Forewarning the casualty of this and other effects will ensure the casualty will be able to tolerate the mask with less anxiety. If the casualty cannot tolerate any form of mask over the face then the two-pronged cannula should be used. This is better than no oxygen at all. Casualties should be encouraged to breathe normally when using therapy masks.

Using a therapy mask on a breathing casualty

1 Turn on the oxygen cylinder.

2 Connect the oxygen mask to the oxygen unit.

3 Turn on the oxygen therapy allowing the oxygen to flow through the mask.

4 Introduce the mask to the casualty explaining the benefits and the effects.

5 Hold the mask to the face, gradually adjusting the elastic around the casualty's head and adjust the malleable nose piece.

6 Observe the casualty's respiration.

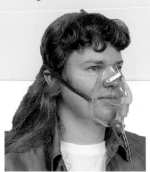

Two-pronged nasal cannula

The two-pronged nasal cannula is devised from plastic tubing
with two plastic tips that sit at the base of the nostrils. It will
deliver oxygen concentration of 30% to 40% with an oxygen
flow rate of 3–5 lpm. Do not use higher flow rates as they
will not increase the delivered oxygen concentration but
will cause irritation of the nasal mucosa. The nasal cannula
is usually well tolerated but it can cause
some soreness around the nostrils and
the maximum oxygen concentration it
will deliver is limited. This device is a
useful means of oxygen delivery when
low to moderate oxygen concentrations
are required. It is mainly used for chronic
airway disease casualties who are
feeling slightly short of breath.
Anyone who has acute shortness
of breath needs high concentrations
of oxygen.

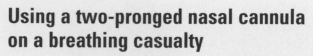

Using a two-pronged nasal cannula on a breathing casualty

1 Turn on the oxygen cylinder.

2 Connect the nasal cannula to the oxygen unit.

3 Turn on the oxygen therapy allowing the oxygen to flow through the nasal cannula.

4 Introduce the nasal cannula to the casualty explaining the benefits and the effects.

5 Observe the casualty's breathing.

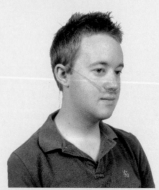

Soft bag resuscitator with oxygen

Soft bag and mask systems are preferred by many first aiders as they can feel the movement of the bag, indicating the condition of the airway, and the presence or absence of breathing. They deliver 100% oxygen to the casualty. Soft bag resuscitators may be used for casualties with severe respiratory distress, unconscious casualties, and those who have been exposed to carbon monoxide inhalation.

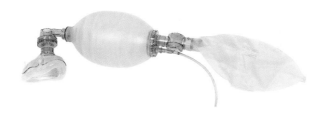

Using a soft bag resuscitator with oxygen on a breathing casualty

1 Attach reservoir bag to soft bag.

2 Attach oxygen to the nipple on the reservoir bag.

3 Turn on oxygen (reservoir bag will inflate at 15 lpm to maintain a full reservoir).

4 Choose appropriate size face mask (adult or child).

5 Place mask over casualty's face (narrow part over bridge of nose). Bring face to the mask to ensure a good seal.

6 Check mask is firmly applied.

7 Hold mask with one hand; as the casualty breathes in, they will automatically receive 100% oxygen until the end of inhalation.

4

Demand valve resuscitator

In breathing casualties inhalation triggers the demand valve and oxygen automatically flows at 100% until inhalation is complete. Expired gases pass into the atmosphere. This is useful for casualties with severe respiratory distress, unconscious casualties and those who have been exposed to carbon monoxide inhalation.

Using a demand valve resuscitator on a breathing casualty

1 Turn on the oxygen cylinder valve anticlockwise. Turn on about one or two full turns.

2 Check contents gauge for adequate supply.

3 Place face mask firmly over nose and mouth ensuring an airtight seal. As the casualty breathes in, the resuscitator will automatically supply 100% oxygen until the end of inhalation.

4 The casualty exhales through the mask—no need to remove the mask.

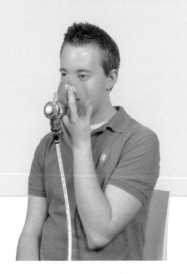

Non-breathing casualty

Demand valve resuscitator

In non-breathing casualties a manual override is used to inflate the lungs. This is operated by depressing a button directly. Excess lung pressure is prevented by a pressure relief valve.

Using a demand valve resuscitator on a non-breathing casualty

1 Kneel at the head of the casualty.

2 Check, clear and open airway.

3 Insert an oropharyngeal airway (if available).

4 Turn on oxygen cylinder valve anticlockwise. Turn on about one or two full turns. Check contents gauge for adequate supply.

5 Choose appropriate size face mask (adult or child).

6 Position face mask over nose, then mouth area, with narrow part of mask between casualty's eyes. Bring face to the mask to ensure a good seal.

7 Ensure that mask fits correctly and does not allow oxygen to escape when used.

8 Check that mask is firmly applied and head tilt is maintained.

9 Press button on the demand valve resuscitator until chest commences to rise, then release and wait until lungs deflate (do not overinflate).

10 Check constantly that equipment is functioning and your technique is correct.

Note: Ensure that you DO NOT overinflate the casualty's lungs. The pressure from a demand valve may cause injury to the lungs if they are overinflated.

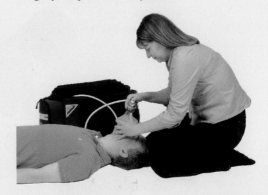

Soft bag resuscitators

Soft bag and mask systems are preferred by many first aiders as they can feel the movement of the bag, indicating the condition of the airway, and the presence or absence of breathing.

Hand powered soft bag resuscitators may be used with or without oxygen connected to the equipment for non-breathing casualties.

Using a soft bag resuscitator with oxygen on a non-breathing casualty

1 Kneel at head of casualty.

2 Check, clear and open airway.

3 Insert an oropharyngeal airway (if available).

4 Attach reservoir bag to soft bag.

5 Attach oxygen to the nipple on the reservoir bag.

6 Turn on oxygen (reservoir bag will inflate at 15 lpm to maintain a full reservoir).

7 Choose appropriate size face mask (adult or child).

8 Place mask over casualty's face (narrow part over bridge of nose). Bring face to the mask to ensure a good seal.

9 Check mask is firmly applied and that head tilt is maintained.

10 Hold mask with one hand; gently squeeze bag with other hand and watch for chest to rise; then release bag.

11 Check constantly that equipment is functioning and your technique is correct.

Using a soft bag resuscitator without oxygen on a non-breathing casualty

1 Kneel at head of casualty.

2 Check, clear and open airway.

3 Insert an oropharyngeal airway (if available).

4 Choose appropriate size face mask (adult or child).

5 Place mask over casualty's face (narrow part over bridge of nose). Bring face to mask to ensure a good seal.

6 Check mask is firmly applied and that head tilt is maintained.

7 Hold mask with one hand; squeeze bag with other hand and watch for chest to rise; then release bag.

8 Check constantly that equipment is functioning and your technique is correct.

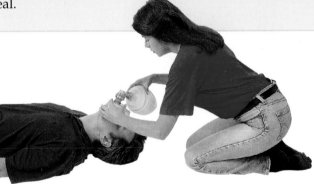

Two first aiders – with oxygen equipment

When CPR is required and two first aiders are present or a second person arrives, and oxygen equipment is available, a changeover of operators when required will minimise fatigue, particularly for the first aider performing compressions. When it is determined that the casualty has no signs of life:

- ensure that an ambulance has been called
- first aider 'one' starts CPR
- first aider 'two' sets up oxygen equipment
- first aider 'one' continues performing compressions
- first aider 'two' takes over breaths using oxygen equipment
- first aider 'one' or 'two' indicates their readiness or need to change every 2 minutes
- change over smoothly with minimal interference to the resuscitation procedure
- ensure the change of operator is done approximately every two minutes to minimise fatigue.

Continue CPR with the use of oxygen until:

- the casualty shows signs of life
- more qualified help arrives
- you both are physically unable to continue.

If the casualty shows signs of life, place casualty in recovery position, provide oxygen therapy, monitor vital signs and manage any injuries while waiting for the ambulance.

Maintaining the airway

Oropharyngeal airway

An oropharyngeal airway is a device used to assist in establishing and maintaining an adequate airway. It may be used in conjunction with a soft bag resuscitator, mechanical resuscitator or face mask on an unconscious, breathing or non-breathing casualty when difficulty is experienced in maintaining an open airway. It should always be inserted with care.

Warning

Only use on an unconscious casualty (it can irritate the back of throat and cause vomiting, coughing and spasm of larynx).

If casualty shows any sign of retching, remove airway device immediately.

Do not use on casualties with tissue trauma to the mouth.

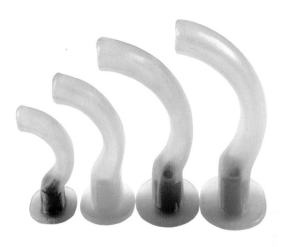

Inserting an oropharyngeal airway

1   Check casualty's airway is clear.

2   Place oropharyngeal airway on casualty's face to check for correct size—tubing should extend from corner of mouth to the tip of the earlobe.

4   Point tip of airway towards roof of casualty's mouth then insert airway approximately 1/3 of its length into casualty's mouth.

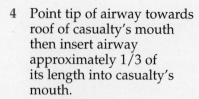

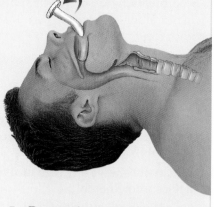

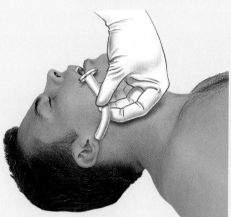

3   To insert, use thumb and index finger crossed to pry the casualty's teeth apart and hold mouth open.

5   Rotate airway over tongue until airway points towards side of casualty's mouth.

6   Gently push airway approximately 2/3 of its length into mouth, rotating so that tip is pointing down the pharynx.

7   Gently push airway further into casualty's mouth until its flange is pressing on lips.

8   Extend casualty's head and, if necessary, apply a jaw thrust to assist in settling oropharyngeal airway into correct position and maintain casualty's airway.

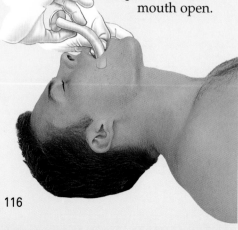

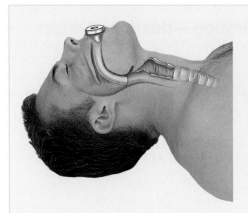

9 If casualty shows any signs of vomiting or rejecting the oropharyngeal airway, remove it immediately.

Note: If spinal injury is suspected, care must be taken with any movement of the head.

Oropharyngeal aspiration

A suction catheter is used to aspirate fluid (e.g. mucus, saliva, vomitus fluid) from the mouth and nose to prevent inhalation of the fluid and to obtain and maintain an unobstructed airway. This should only be carried out on an unconscious casualty otherwise the casualty will gag involuntarily. Prior to any suction, the oropharyngeal airway must be removed.

Oropharyngeal aspiration—flexible catheter ('Y' suction tube)

1 Connect appropriate size 'Y' suction catheter to end of suction tubing.

2 Determine maximum length of catheter by measuring distance from corner of casualty's nose to the earlobe (place catheter against face).

3 Turn suction source on.

4 Open casualty's mouth with crossed fingers technique *(see p. 116)*.

5 Insert catheter to appropriate depth with 'Y' piece open.

6 Aspirate by blocking 'Y' piece on catheter with a finger and rotating catheter continuously during removal—aspirate for a maximum of 5 seconds at any one time.

7 Allow casualty to breathe oxygen, or ventilate casualty.

8 Ensure aspiration bowl does not fill beyond 2/3 full.

Note: DO NOT leave suction turned on unnecessarily as it wastes oxygen at approximately 20 lpm.

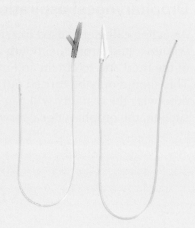

Oropharyngeal aspiration—rigid suction tube (Yankauer sucker)

1 Connect Yankauer suction catheter to suction tubing.

2 Turn suction source on.

3 Open casualty's mouth with crossed finger technique (see p. 116).

4 Hold suction-head handle by cradling it in curved fingers of one hand, leaving thumb free.

5 Insert suction tube tip into direct-view area of pharynx without open tip of suction-head being blocked (the curve matches mouth and pharynx).

6 Aspirate casualty by blocking hole if present in tube (adjacent to suction handle) with thumb of hand holding suction-head handle. Aspirate for maximum of 5 seconds.

7 Withdraw suction-head slowly.

8 Ventilate casualty or return supplemental oxygen therapy device.

9 Ensure aspiration bowl (suction bottle) does not fill beyond 2/3 full.

Note: DO NOT leave suction turned on unnecessarily as it wastes oxygen at approximately 20 lpm.

Oropharyngeal aspiration—straight catheter

1 Connect appropriate size suction catheter to end of suction tubing.

2 Determine maximum length of catheter by measuring distance from corner of nose to earlobe (place catheter against face).

3 Open casualty's mouth with crossed finger technique (see p. 116).

4 Insert catheter to appropriate depth.

5 Aspirate by squeezing the handle of manual suction unit with one hand. Rotate and withdraw the catheter with the other hand

continuously during removal—aspirate for maximum of 5 seconds at any one time.

6 Allow casualty to breathe oxygen, or ventilate casualty.

7 Ensure aspiration bowl does not fill beyond 2/3 full.

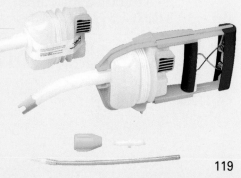

Defibrillation

A defibrillator is used to treat Sudden Cardiac Arrest (SCA), a condition that occurs when the heart unexpectedly stops pumping.

Cardiopulmonary resuscitation can maintain the blood flow and keep the blood oxygenated, but SCA is usually caused by fibrillation, a disturbance of the electrical activity in the heart's ventricular muscle, or larger pumping chamber. It causes the heart to quiver or 'fibrillate' in a disordered way. The electrical disruption prevents the heart from pumping blood around the body effectively causing the heart to stop beating, leading to a cardiac arrest.

It is fatal if the casualty is not resuscitated quickly. With the use of a defibrillator, an electric shock can be delivered to stop the fibrillation. Providing the heart is well oxygenated and the chemistry surrounding the heart is within acceptable limits, the heart should start beating again. This electrical shock must be delivered by a defibrillator.

A sudden cardiac arrest can occur in the young or old, male or female – anywhere, at any time, and there may be no warning signs or symptoms. There are two main groups of cardiac arrest casualties.

1   A cardiac event is the cause of sudden cardiac arrest.
2   Sudden cardiac arrest is secondary to non-cardiac causes e.g. drowning or blood loss from trauma.

Casualties in the first of these groups are usually conscious until sudden cardiac arrest occurs and are more likely to have the arrest reversed.

Casualties in the second group can be effectively treated only if the underlying cause is dealt with.

Not all abnormal rhythms after cardiac arrest are reversible. If the heart does not have any electrical activity there is no benefit in giving defibrillation. The AED will determine accurately if the heart will benefit from a shock. Sometimes the underlying problem/disease causing the SCA is not survivable despite any accessible care. CPR should be continued until expert help arrives or you are unable to continue.

Use of defibrillators

Automated external defibrillators (AEDs) were originally designed for adults, but some manufacturers now offer suitable pads for application to children that reduce the adult size shock. Adhesive defibrillator pads are attached to the casualty (*see p. 123*). Signs of life are checked and if none are present, the machine will analyse the casualty's heart rhythm automatically. The AED makes a diagnosis of the heart rhythm and advises the operator whether to shock the casualty or not by displaying messages on a screen and by voice prompts.

The AED voice prompt will direct that everyone stands clear of the casualty and instruct the operator to press the 'Shock' button. The shock button is only activated if a shockable rhythm is diagnosed or, depending on the AED, will automatically shock the casualty.

Before taking a defibrillator for use in the field, make sure you have:

*   1 disposable towel
*   disposable razor designed for removing chest hair
*   1 pair dressing shears/blunt nosed scissors
*   disposable gloves
*   2 defibrillator pads (store in a cool environment and keep flat)
*   pocket mask or face shield.

Care in the use of defibrillators

Always ensure that everyone is clear of the casualty during analysis and before discharging the shock.

- Ensure oxygen output is not directed towards the area of defibrillation, or have oxygen equipment switched off.

- Ensure mobile phones and two-way radios are switched off, or at least 2 metres away.

- NEVER defibrillate in a moving vehicle.

- Regularly check defibrillation equipment.

- DO NOT fold self-adhesive pads.

- Regularly have the equipment serviced by authorised agents.

- Clean the defibrillator after use with a soft cloth.

Note: It is safe to defibrillate a casualty on either a wet or metal surface provided care is taken to ensure that no one is touching the casualty when the shock button is pressed.

Defibrillating a casualty

1 Follow **DRABCD**.

2 Establish that casualty has no signs of life (unresponsive, not breathing and not moving).

3 **Call 000** for an ambulance—ask bystander if present.

4 Commence CPR, and continue during following steps.

5 Expose casualty's chest.

6 Remove any medication patches, check for pacemaker or defibrillator implant (look for scar between the collar bone and top of the breast (either left or right side of chest).

7 Wipe chest to ensure it is dry—if chest is hairy clip with scissors or use razor.

8 Depending on the type of defibrillator either, attach cables to defibrillator pads or pull handle on the device to access pads.

9 Attach pads to casualty's chest:

- one pad to casualty's right chest wall—below collarbone (ensure pad adheres to skin)

- one pad to casualty's left chest wall—below left nipple (ensure pad adheres to skin).

Note: *If implant is identified, place pad at least 5 cm away from site— do not place pad on top of pacemaker or implant site.*

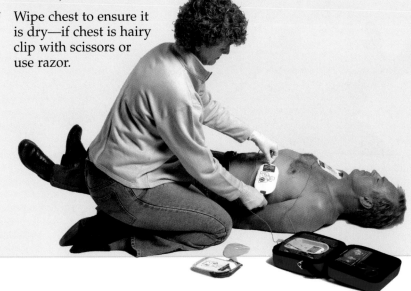

10 Press 'On' button firmly (if relevant to model of defibrillator).

11 Stop CPR.

12 Make sure no one is touching the casualty.

13 Follow machine's instructions (voice prompts).

14 If no shock advised, follow voice prompts.

15 If shock advised:

- ensure it is safe to defibrillate
- no one touch the casualty
- press the 'Shock' button or stand clear for automatic AED to shock
- follow voice prompts.

16 If the casualty responds to defibrillation, continue CPR until the casualty pushes the rescuer away or it is clear that there are signs of life.

Note: DO NOT remove defibrillator pads (even if casualty is conscious).

17 If the area is not safe or you are unsure, turn AED off.

Defibrillation with children

In children, non-cardiac causes of cardiac arrest such as drowning or suffocation are more likely to occur. In such cases there is unlikely to be heart electrical activity, and defibrillation is therefore unlikely to be of assistance. However, there are a number of AEDs approved for use in Australia, and whilst each one is slightly different, they all follow the same basic approach as outlined below. Users should follow the visual and/or voice prompts of the particular AED being used.

A standard AED may be used on a child eight years or older (over approximately 25kg) and in cardiac arrest.

For children under 8 years, or less than 25kg who have no signs of life, use child/infant pads. If a child appears to be older than 8 years or larger than 25kg use adult pads. Do not delay treatment to determine the child's exact age or weight.

Note: *Almost all infants and young children who have no signs of life are more likely to be in respiratory arrest. Therefore, CPR should not be interrupted during the preparation for defibrillation.*

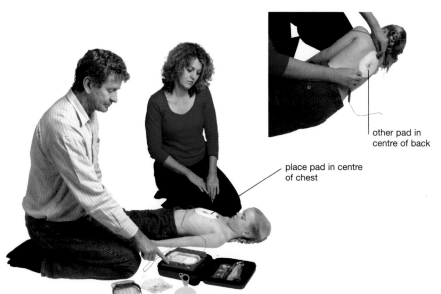

other pad in centre of back

place pad in centre of chest

4

State of Readiness

Automated External Defibrillators are very easy to maintain and have extensive automatic self-test features which eliminate the need for any manual calibration. The AED has been manufactured to perform automatic self-testing daily/weekly and monthly, which saves time, improves testing consistency and minimises unnecessary battery expenditure.

It is important that the Automated External Defibrillator is checked weekly and maintained in a continual 'state of readiness' to ensure that it is 'ready' for use in an emergency. Regular checking and maintaining of the defibrillator and consumables should be done in accordance with manufacturer's instructions and checklists for the particular AED model.

The weekly check includes:
1   Checking that the green Ready Light/Indicator is flashing/visible. If not, consult manual for recommended action.
2   Checking supplies and accessories for damage and expiration dating. Replace any used, damaged or expired items.
3   Checking the outside of the AED for cracks or other signs of damage. If you see signs of damage, contact your local branch of St John Ambulance Australia or manufacturer for technical support. Ensure the defibrillator pads are stored flat and in a cool area.

If the defibrillator is dirty or contaminated, the outside of your AED and the case can be cleaned with a soft cloth dampened with either:
• soapy water
• chlorine bleach (2 tablespoons per litre of water)
• ammonia-based cleaners.

Note: *Do not use isopropyl (rubbing) alcohol, strong solvents such as acetone of acetone-based cleaners, abrasive materials, or enzymatic cleaners on the AED. Do not immerse the AED in fluids or allow fluids to spill onto it. Do not sterilise the defibrillator or its accessories (refer to manufacturers instructions).*

5

Shock

What is shock?

If the circulatory system fails, insufficient oxygen reaches the vital organs and the tissues. This triggers a series of responses that leads to the condition known as shock.

What causes shock?

Shock is caused by a lack of circulating blood volume. The volume is too low to meet the body's needs and to remove the waste products. Shock is caused by:

- the heart failing
- bleeding
- vomiting and diarrhoea
- burns
- pain
- trauma
- infections
- allergic reactions.

A casualty's physical injuries may not appear to be severe but may result in life-threatening consequences associated with shock.

If the volume of blood circulating around the body is reduced, the cells quickly become depleted of oxygen. This causes shock at the cellular level and produces the signs of shock in the whole body. This can be particularly serious in infants, children and the elderly. A spinal cord injury can also result in shock.

Shock in infants and children, as in adults, is a life-threatening condition that may occur as a result of a serious injury or illness, particularly when there is severe bleeding or fluid loss. It is a progressive condition involving the collapse of the circulatory system, and may lead to death.

Shock is not always readily apparent immediately after an injury. The signs and symptoms develop gradually and depend on the severity of the injury. Shock also depends on whether fluid loss continues and on the effectiveness of management of the injury. Gastroenteritis can be particularly serious in infants and young children. If a child loses a lot of fluid as a result of vomiting or diarrhoea, there is a loss of blood volume which can mean there is insufficient blood to transport oxygen to the tissues. This leads to shock.

Immediately after injury, there may be little evidence of shock. It is important that you treat the injury or illness which is causing the shock as well as treating the shock and the person as a whole. The signs and symptoms may develop progressively, depending on:

- the severity of the injury
- continuation of fluid loss
- effectiveness of management.

SIGNS AND SYMPTOMS OF INITIAL SHOCK

- pale face, fingernails and lips
- cold, clammy skin
- faintness or dizziness
- nausea
- anxiety.

SIGNS AND SYMPTOMS OF SEVERE SHOCK

- restlessness
- thirst
- weak, rapid pulse
- shallow, fast breathing
- drowsiness, confusion or unconsciousness
- extremities become bluish in colour—this is a late sign and the person is very sick.

Note: If the casualty has dark skin or skin colour is obscured due to e.g. severe burns, soot, face pain, check colour of skin on the inside of lower eyelid or inside lower lip.

TRY NOT to leave a casualty suffering from shock unattended—send someone else (if available) to make the call for the ambulance.

Management of shock

1   Follow **DRABCD** and manage injuries such as severe bleeding.

2   Reassure the casualty.

3   **Call 000** for an ambulance.

4   Raise the casualty's legs (unless fractured or a snake bite) above the level of the heart—place head flat on floor.

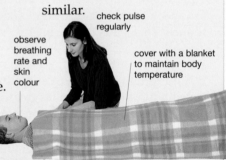

observe breathing rate and skin colour

similar.

check pulse regularly

cover with a blanket to maintain body temperature

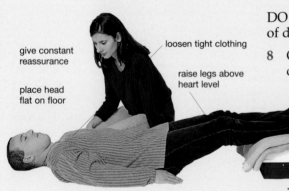

give constant reassurance

place head flat on floor

loosen tight clothing

raise legs above heart level

DO NOT use any source of direct heat.

8   Give small amounts of clear fluid (preferably water) frequently to the conscious casualty who does not have abdominal trauma and unlikely to require an operation in the immediate future.

5   Treat any wound or burn and immobilise any fractures.

6   Loosen any tight clothing at neck chest and waist.

7   Maintain casualty's body warmth with a blanket or

9   Monitor and record breathing, pulse and skin colour at regular intervals.

10 Place the casualty in recovery position if there is breathing difficulty, the casualty becomes unconscious or is likely to vomit.

6

Infection control

Disease transmission

The spread of infection requires a source of infecting micro-organisms, a potential host and a means of transmission. Infection may be transmitted via breathing, coughing, touching, eating, or body penetration. This latter may occur following wounding or as a result of sexual transmission. The same organism can be transmitted by more than one route.

Best practice first aid will ensure infection control. Under very rare conditions transmission of disease can occur in the first aid context. Such diseases include colds and respiratory viral diseases. There are extremely rare instances of tuberculosis (TB) and hepatitis being contracted by ambulance personnel or first aiders working in the pre-hospital environment. There are no proven cases of HIV (Aids) being contracted by such workers.

Infection control is achieved by protecting both the casualty and the first aider from the transmission of:

- blood and bodily fluids (e.g. saliva, vomit, pus, urine, faeces)
- infected hypodermic needles or sharp objects
- droplets (e.g. nasal, throat or airway secretions).

Ensuring good hygiene practices is extremely important in preventing disease transmission. Unless the first aider takes all necessary precautions, disease transmission may occur to the casualty or be passed on to the first aider. Therefore, it is important to assume that every situation is potentially infectious. First aiders should check with their general practitioner that their vaccinations are current (particularly Hepatitis B) as per the current *Australian Immunisation Handbook*.

Standard precautions

'Standard precautions' are the words used to describe practices required to achieve infection control. Standard precautions are the basis on which all current first aid is administered to casualties, regardless of their perceived or actual infectious status.

Standard precautions include good hygiene practices, particularly washing and drying hands before and after contact with a casualty and may include wearing personal protective equipment such as gloves, face masks/shields, eye protection and protective clothing as appropriate.

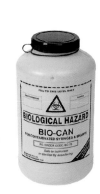

In addition to personal protective equipment and hand washing, appropriate handling and disposal of 'sharps' and other clinical waste which may contaminated or infectious, should be followed.

Clinical waste includes:

- used 'sharps'
- any human tissue or fluids, including material or solutions containing free-flowing blood.
- dressings contaminated by blood or body fluids.

Container for used 'sharps' (e.g. syringe, blood-testing needle)

Respiratory hygiene/coughing etiquette

Respiratory secretions may be passed from person to person by coughing, by hand-to-hand, hand-to-nose, hand-to-eye or hand-to-mouth contact. All people with signs or symptoms of a respiratory infection, regardless of presumed cause should:

- cover the nose/mouth when coughing or sneezing with a tissue or cough and sneeze into the elbow fold
- use tissues to contain respiratory secretions
- spit into tissue if spitting in necessary
- dispose of tissues in the nearest rubbish bin after use
- wash their hands thoroughly after contact with respiratory secretions and contaminated objects or materials
- offer a surgical mask for casualties to wear if they are being treated in a first aid facility and coughing
- encourage coughing persons to sit at least 1 metre away from others in common waiting areas.

If available, a pocket mask or face shield should be used when undertaking mouth-to-mouth resuscitation.

Handwashing and protective equipment

Handwashing is the most important measure in preventing the spread of infection (germs). Hands should be washed before and after contact with a casualty and after activities likely to cause contamination.

Protective gloves should be worn when it is likely that your hands will be contaminated with blood or body fluid, or come into contact with mucous membranes.

Other personal protective equipment such as face masks, eye protection, resuscitation masks or shields should be used as appropriate.

Before first aid:

- Wash hands thoroughly with soap and warm running water and dry thoroughly, preferably with a paper towel and dispose.
- If soap and water are not available, clean hands with antiseptic 'wipes', then apply an alcohol-based liquid or gel.
- Cover any exposed wounds with a waterproof dressing.
- Do not touch infected wounds or potentially infected material (e.g. dressings) with your bare hands.
- Put on disposable protective gloves. If you have an allergy or sensitivity to latex, use nitrile gloves.
- Use other personal protective equipment if required.
- If your gloves tear while giving first aid, take them off straight away, wash and dry hands, then put on a new pair of gloves.

After first aid:

- Dispose of any dressing contaminated with blood or body fluids, and used gloves inside two plastic bags tied securely and placed in the general refuse or garbage disposal system.
- If a 'yellow bag system' is available, place any such contaminated dressings in these; they must then be disposed of in a special 'contaminated waste' system (such as a hospital).
- Remove gloves without touching the outside surface of gloves with your bare hands (see p. 136).
- Wash hands thoroughly with soap and warm running water and dry thoroughly.

If work surfaces have become contaminated:

- Appropriate personal protective clothing (e.g. eye protection, plastic apron, mask and protective gloves) should be worn when cleaning blood or other body fluid spills.
- Clean contaminated surfaces with detergent and water— use a 10% bleach solution if surface is contaminated with blood or body fluids.

- When cleaning large spills (greater than 10 cm), caution is required as the risk of a splash is very high. Special granular sachets can be used to soak up fluid and left in place for 10 minutes, then swept up and disposed of. If granular sachets are not available use 10% bleach solution. The surface should then be mopped with detergent and water.

- Wash and disinfect resuscitation masks in warm water and detergent, rinse and allow them to dry. Then soak in a 10% solution of bleach (in well-ventilated area) for not less than 10 minutes. Rinse masks in cold running water and air dry in a clean environment.

Note: Valves and filters in pocket masks are 'single use only'— dispose of in the general refuse after use.

How to remove gloves

All gloves used in first aid are disposable. Once gloves are used in first aid, they are contaminated and can be a source of infection.

They must be taken off without touching the outside surface and where possible, hands washed and dried immediately.

slide fingers under the cuff of second glove (i.e. inside the glove)

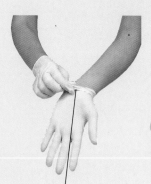

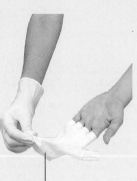

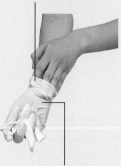

grasp the upper outside of the cuff of one of the gloves

pull glove off hand and fingers, turning glove inside out

pull glove off hand and fingers, turning glove inside out

place gloves in plastic bag and seal

wash hands with soap and running water

Blood and needle-stick accidents

Correct management of exposure to blood, or body fluids contaminated with blood and needle-stick or 'sharps' injuries will reduce to zero any potential for infection with Human Immunodeficiency Virus (HIV), Hepatitis B Virus (HBV), Hepatitis C Virus (HCV) or other blood-borne infectious agents.

Exposure to risk of infection has occurred when:

- a needle contaminated with blood or body fluid has penetrated the skin
- a wound has been caused by an instrument contaminated with blood or body fluid
- a wound or skin lesion (dermatitis) has been contaminated with blood or body fluid
- there has been mucous membrane or eye contact with blood or body fluid.

Any item (e.g. blood, body fluid, 'sharp') considered to be a potential source of infection should be safely contained. The contaminated item should be kept for testing, if required. Blood contaminated clothing should be removed.

Any first aider who has been exposed to any of the above risks of infection must seek medical advice within hours of such an exposure.

Immediate care of the exposed site

If the skin is involved (e.g. needle-stick), wash the area well with soap and water (an antiseptic such as povidine-iodine could also be applied). DO NOT make the affected area bleed. If water is not available, clean the area with hand wipes followed by an alcohol-based liquid or gel if available.

Eyes, if contaminated or splashed with blood or body fluids, should be irrigated gently but thoroughly with copious running water or normal saline. At least 5 minutes washing is advised. The eyes must be kept open during this process.

When the mouth is involved contaminated fluid should be spat out and the mouth rinsed thoroughly with water several times.

Referral and risk assessment following unprotected blood or body fluid exposure

The infectious status of the source individual is almost always unknown. All casualties should be regarded as potentially infectious. Any contaminated first aider must seek referral and counsel by a medical practitioner or health care worker with experience in infection control or occupational health. Alternatively, the affected person should be referred immediately to the nearest hospital for assessment and evaluation of potential disease transmission. Only a very small proportion of accidental exposures to blood result in an infection from a blood-borne virus (i.e. HIV or HBV).

Confidentiality and documentation

All details relating to the circumstances and the potential source of a risk exposure must be kept confidential. Information should only be provided to health care professionals who are involved in the care process. The incident must be comprehensively documented and stored appropriately (see p. 411).

7

Basic first aid equipment

First aid kits

A first aid kit is a necessity for every first aider—indeed for every home, your car and in the workplace. It contains the bandages, dressings, pads, gloves and other items needed to deal with any situation.

All open wounds need some type of covering to help control bleeding, to prevent and minimise bacterial contamination and possible infection. Dressings and bandages are the main items used by the first aider. Different types of dressings and bandages are used, in varying ways, depending on the type and severity of the injury and the materials available.

Other items may be used for dressing a wound—pads to help absorb blood or to give extra protection, swabs for cleaning, tape to keep dressings in place, and a range of sundry items such as scissors and towels.

Knowing what each item is used for and how it is used is very important. The way in which you use and apply these materials will vary with the type of injury and where the injury is located on the body.

The contents of first aid kits used in the workplace are covered by regulations in each State or Territory.

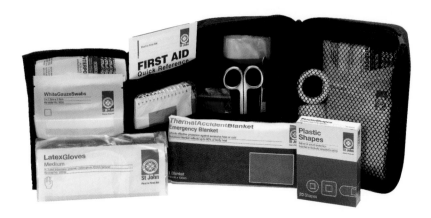

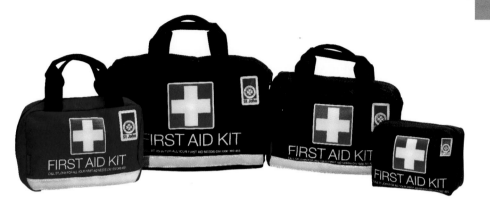

It is important to ensure that you regularly check the contents of your first aid kit to make sure they are clean, packets are properly sealed, expiry dates have not been exceeded, and that you have replaced any previously used items.

Although it is safer to use sterile bandages and dressings, there will be emergencies when you will not have a first aid kit immediately to hand. You will then have to use whatever materials you can find. St John offers a large range of first aid kits, services and products.

Remember

Check the contents of your first aid kit after every use and immediately replace any used and out-of-date items.

Items a first aid kit contains

The following is a list of items and their uses that may be included in your first aid kit:

Wound dressings

- 10 cm x 10 cm non-adherent dressings:
  - for use when you don't want the bandage to stick to the wound (e.g. burns, weeping or oozing wounds)
- No. 13 wound dressing:
  - to control bleeding and protect minor wounds
- No. 14 wound dressing:
  - to control bleeding and protect moderate wounds
- No. 15 wound dressing:
  - to control bleeding and protect major wounds
- Adhesive shapes:
  - for small cuts and abrasions.

Pads

- 9 cm x 20 cm combine pads:
  - for padding of major injuries
  - for placing over non-adherent dressings
- Eye pads:
  - for covering wounded eyes.

Swabs

- 7.5 cm x 7.5 cm x 3 cm gauze swabs:
  - for cleaning wounds and surrounding areas
- Alcohol swabs:
  - for cleaning first aider's hands.

Bandages

- Triangular bandages:
  - for emergency dressings
  - as slings to support upper arm
- 10 cm crepe or conforming bandages:
  - for pressure immobilisation after snakebite and some other bites and stings
  - to bind large/medium dressings in place

- 7.5 cm conforming bandages:
  - to bind medium dressings in place
- 5 cm conforming bandages:
  - to bind medium/small dressings in place.

Other items

- Roll of adhesive tape—at least 24 mm wide and 2.5 m long:
  - to secure light dressings
- disposable hand towels:
  - For general cleaning—not wounds
- pair of stainless steel scissors:
  - To cut dressings, bandages
- Blunt-nosed shears:
  - to cut away clothing
- 30 ml saline eyewash:
  - for eye irrigation and wound cleaning
- Safety pins:
  - to secure bandages and slings
- Stingose® gel:
  - to soothe irritation of insect bites and stings
- Medium plastic bags:
  - various uses (e.g. to make icepacks, carry water, seal an open chest wound, store dressings)
- Stainless steel tweezers:
  - for removing splinters
- Thermo blanket:
  - for protection against the elements, to prevent loss of body heat
- Note pad and pencil:
  - for recording times and details
- Disposable gloves:
  - to assist in preventing cross infection.

Wound dressings

Dressings should be sterile or clean and placed directly
on a wound to:

- absorb blood and other body fluids
- keep the wound clean
- help protect the wound from infection
- reduce pain.

General principles for applying dressings

1 Wash hands before
applying clean disposable
gloves.

2 Use a sterile dressing that
extends about 2 cm past
the edges of the wound.

3 Do not touch the surface
that will contact the
wound.

4 If the wound is minor,
clean with sterile or clean
water before applying the
dressing.

5 Replace at least once a
day any dressing which
becomes wet or soiled.

6 Wash your hands after
removing gloves.

Adhesive dressings

Adhesive dressings are generally used for minor wounds. They have an absorbent pad attached to an adhesive strip or backing. They come in many shapes and sizes and may be packaged individually within packets or be available as a continuous strip.

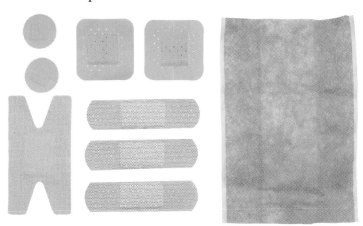

Non-adherent dressings

Non-adherent dressings can be used with any injury, but are especially useful for burns and abrasions, where the injury is to the surface of the skin and it is important to prevent blood and fluids sticking to the dressing. Because they do not adhere to the skin, they can usually be removed easily.

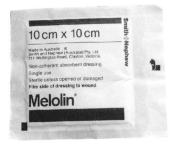

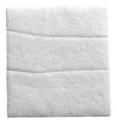

Combine and BPC dressings

Combine and BPC dressings comprise a bandage, pad and dressing in one unit and are used for large or deep wounds. Because they are made of layers of gauze and cotton wool, their bulk is useful for controlling bleeding and for absorbing discharge.

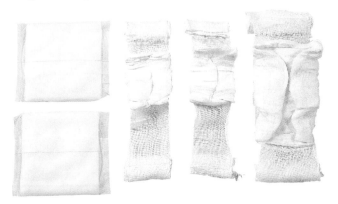

Apply a combine or BPC dressing

1   Hold an end of bandage in each hand and position pad on wound.

2   Wrap shorter end around limb or trunk of body to hold in place.

3   Wrap longer end over dressing until covered.

4   Tie ends with a reef knot.

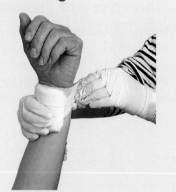

Bandages

A bandage is any material used to wrap or cover a wound.

Bandages are used to:
* keep dressings in place
* control bleeding
* protect a wound from dirt and infection
* give support and pain relief
* restrict movement
* minimise swelling
* immobilise fractures—usually with splints.
* keep splints in position.

Triangular bandages

Triangular bandages can be used as dressings, pads, padding or slings. If used to bandage a wound, they should be secured with a reef knot. They can be made by cutting a one metre square piece of cloth diagonally into two triangular pieces. If the triangular bandage is too large for your needs, fold it in half.

Triangular bandages can be folded and used as a pad. Pads are thick and bulky and primarily used to:
* help control bleeding
* absorb blood and other secretions
* help prevent infection
* protect sensitive areas
* give extra padding.

Fold a triangular bandage to use as a pad

1   Place point of triangle down on base.

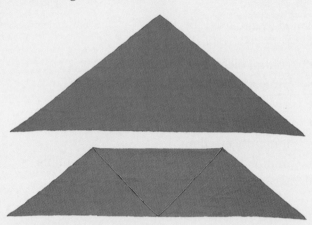

2   Fold in half to make a broad bandage.

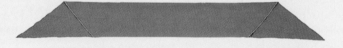

3   Fold in half again to make a narrow bandage.

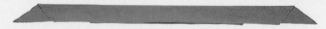

4   Bring ends to middle (do twice).

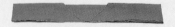

5   Fold in half again to make a pad.

Note: Bandages can be folded this way for storage.

Triangular bandages can be used to secure a dressing
or padding at the knee or elbow when a roller bandage
is not available.

Apply a triangular bandage to knee

1 Fold a narrow hem across
base of bandage.

2 Place the centre of base on
leg below kneecap with the
point towards top of leg.

3 Take bandage ends around
the leg crossing over at
back and bring to front.

4 Tie above kneecap using
a reef knot.

5 Fold the rest of bandage
down and secure with
tape or tuck in.

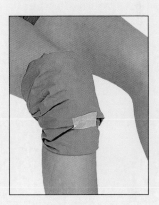

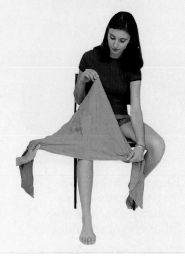

While a triangular bandage can be used to hold a dressing
in place on the head, or to bandage a foot or hand, these tasks
can be more easily accomplished using an elastic (conforming)
roller bandage *(see p. 155)*.

Slings

The St John sling

The St John sling supports the elbow and prevents arm from pulling on an injured shoulder or collarbone.

Apply a St John sling

1   Place casualty's arm naturally by the side, elbow bent (if able) with fingers pointed to the opposite shoulder).

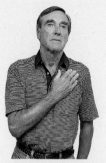

2   Drape an open triangular bandage over forearm, with point past elbow and one end over uninjured shoulder.

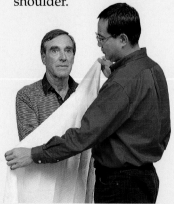

3   Supporting the arm—tuck the base (long side) of bandage under hand and forearm and around elbow.

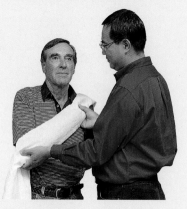

4   Bring the lower end up diagonally across casualty's back to meet other end at shoulder.

5   Gently adjust height of sling.

6   Tie ends as close to fingers as possible.

7   Tuck the point firmly in between forearm and bandage to support elbow.

8 When you are sure sling is firm, secure the fold with a safety pin or tape.

9 Check the circulation by applying gentle pressure to a fingernail—normal colour should return rapidly to the nail when you stop pressing it.

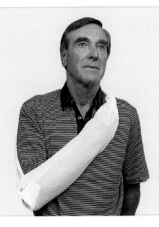

Collar and cuff sling

The collar and cuff sling is a useful sling for a fracture of the upper arm or an injured hand.

Apply a collar and cuff sling

1 Make a clove hitch, using a narrow bandage.

2 Put the loops over the wrist of the injured arm.

3 Gently elevate the injured arm against the casualty's chest.

4 Tie bandage ends together around neck using reef knot positioned in hollow of collarbone.

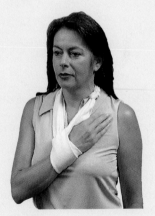

The full arm sling

The full arm sling is used to support an injured forearm and/or wrist.

Apply a full arm sling

1 Place an open triangular bandage between chest and injured arm, with one end of the base length over uninjured shoulder and the other end pointing towards the ground—point of bandage is near elbow.

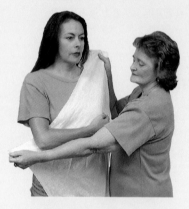

2 Bring the injured forearm slightly above the horizontal position.

3 Tie lower end of bandage to upper end in the hollow above collarbone on injured side (use a reef knot).

4 Carefully arrange bandage so the fingers are showing.

5 Bring the point of bandage to the front of elbow of injured arm and secure with a safety pin.

6 Check the circulation by applying gentle pressure to a fingernail (normal colour should return rapidly to the nail when you stop pressing it).

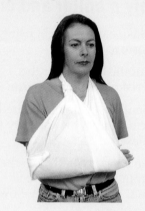

Improvised slings

If there is no bandage available to make a sling, the casualty's clothing can be used to provide support. You can turn up the bottom of a jacket or shirt, use a belt or a tie, or place the hand inside a partially buttoned up shirt or jacket.

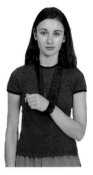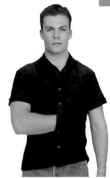

Knots

The reef knot

The reef knot is used to tie bandages because it does not slip, can be untied quite easily, lies flat and does not dig into the wound.

1   Take an end of the bandage in each hand.

2   Place the right-hand end over the left-hand end.

3   Turn it under and bring to the top so that it is now on the left.

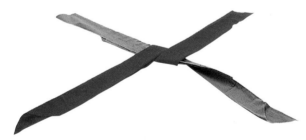

4   Place the new left-hand end over the new right-hand end.

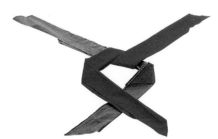

5   Turn it under and bring to the top so that it is now on the right.

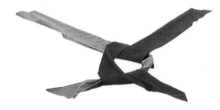

6   Tighten by pulling evenly on both ends.

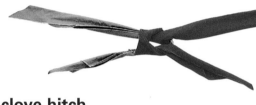

The clove hitch

The clove hitch is used to make a collar and cuff sling. Use a narrow triangular bandage, tie or belt at least 1 metre long.

1   Make two loops (the ends go in opposite directions).

2   Place your hands under the loops and bring them together.

3   Slide the loops over casualty's arm and position them at wrist.

4   Tie the ends around neck (reef knot in hollow of collarbone).

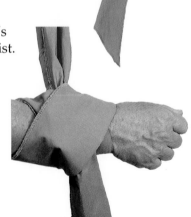

Roller bandages

Roller bandages can be elastic (conforming) or non-elastic. They are made from long strips of material (cotton, gauze, elastic or synthetic) and come in varying widths. They can be used to wrap around parts of the body that are fairly straight, such as the wrist or fingers, to apply pressure to control bleeding, to keep dressings in place and to support an injured part.

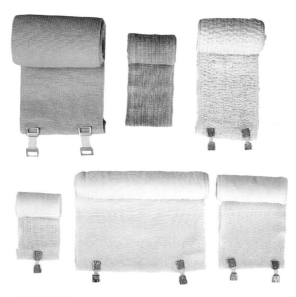

Roller bandages

Roller bandages can be used to bandage the elbow, knee, hand or foot. When applying a roller bandage to the elbow or knee, make alternate turns above and below the joint (figure of eight pattern). Elastic roller bandages are usually used for sprains and other musculoskeletal injuries where an even pressure is necessary to support the joint or to reduce or prevent swelling.

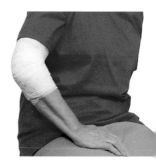

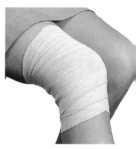

Apply a roller bandage to the hand or foot

1 Secure the 'tail' of bandage with one turn around wrist or ankle.

2 Bring the next turn in a diagonal from wrist or ankle to little finger or toe.

3 Take bandage across palm of hand or sole of foot and back to wrist or ankle.

4 Continue to use a figure of eight pattern to cover hand or foot—leave fingers or toes exposed.

5 Make final turn around wrist or ankle and secure with adhesive tape or tuck in.

6 Check circulation to ensure bandage is not too tight (*see p. 193*).

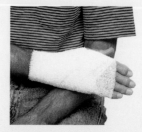

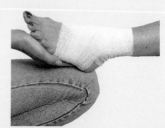

Apply a roller bandage to the arm

1 Place 'tail' end of bandage below the wound, keeping roll of bandage uppermost.

2 Make one full turn over limb to hold 'tail' in place.

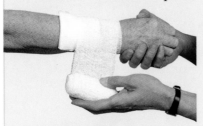

3 Bandage along limb in a spiral fashion, each turn of the bandage covering two-thirds of the one before.

OR

Bandage along limb using a figure of eight pattern.

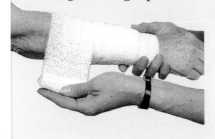

4 Fasten the end with adhesive tape, use clip provided, or tuck in.

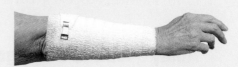

5 Check circulation and adjust bandage if necessary (see p. 193).

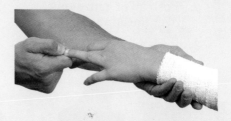

Tubular gauze bandages

Tubular gauze bandages are made of seamless stretch gauze tubing and are used to bandage fingers and toes. Tubular bandages are applied with a specially designed applicator or are stretched by hand to cover and retain a dressing.

Apply a tubular bandage

1 Cut a piece of bandage approximately three times as long as finger to be bandaged.

2 Push all of gauze tube over the applicator.

3 Push applicator over the finger.

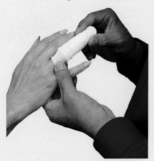

4 Hold end of tubular bandage at base of finger.

5 Pull applicator off finger.

6 Rotate applicator once or twice to twist gauze bandage at end of finger.

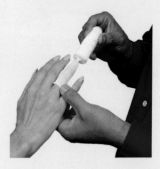

7 Push applicator over finger to apply second layer of bandage.

8 Secure end with tape.

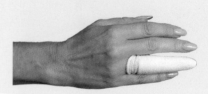

Cold compress

A cold compress relieves pain and swelling by reducing the flow of blood to the injured area. It is usually left on the injury for 15 minutes at a time (as in RICE) and is changed whenever necessary to maintain the same level of coldness. It is usually left uncovered but can be secured with a gauze bandage or some other open-weave material.

Making a cold compress

Use a cloth wrung out in cold water—needs replacing every 10 minutes.	Use a bag of frozen vegetables wrapped in a light wet towel to protect the injury.	Use ice sealed in a plastic bag, two-thirds full of water, wrapped in a light wet towel.

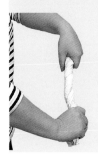 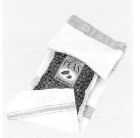 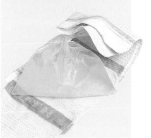

RICE management

R REST the casualty and the injured part.

I ICEPACKS (cold compress) wrapped in a wet cloth may be applied to the injury—for 15 minutes every 2 hours for 24 hours, then for 15 minutes every 4 hours for 24 hours.

C COMPRESSION BANDAGES, such as elastic bandages, should be firmly applied to extend well beyond the injury.

E ELEVATE the injured part.

Pressure immobilisation bandage

A pressure immobilisation bandage applies pressure over wide areas of a limb. It compresses the tiny lymphatic vessels which carry most venoms.

A pressure immobilisation bandage, together with splinting, is an effective form of management because the pressure over the bite area and limb slows the rate at which venom enters the circulation and is transported around the body. This delays the general effects of the venom.

Pressure immobilisation is used for bites and stings from the following:

- snakes
- funnel-web spider
- mouse spider
- blue-ringed octopus
- cone shell.

Note: For an allergic reaction to a bite or sting on a limb, apply a pressure immobilisation bandage.

DO NOT use pressure immobilisation for any of the following, **unless** the casualty has a known allergy to the venom:

- red-back, white-tailed or recluse spider bite
- bee, wasp or ant stings
- tick bite
- bluebottle or Pacific man-of-war stings
- venomous fish stings (e.g. stonefish, stingray).

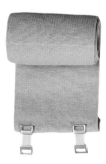

Apply a pressure immobilisation bandage

Use crepe or conforming roller bandage (about 10-15 cm wide)—otherwise pantyhose or other material.

1   Immediately apply a firm roller bandage starting just above the fingers or toes and moving upwards as far as can be reached up the limb.

2   Apply tightly—without stopping blood supply to limb.

3   Immobilise the limb using a splint—secure with second bandage.

4   Check at fingers or toes for circulation (blood supply).

5   Keep the casualty and the limb at rest.

6   DO NOT remove splint or bandage once applied.

Note: DO NOT allow the casualty to move.

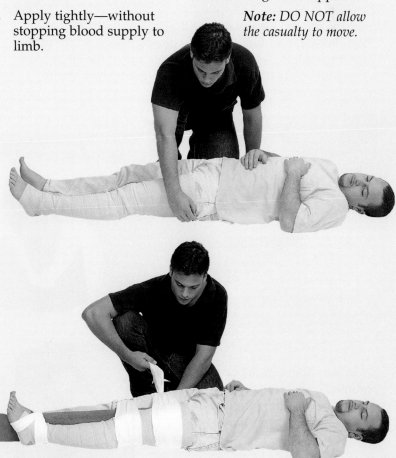

Splints

Splints are used to immobilise and support a limb or injured part of the body. This is particularly important if the casualty has to be moved.

Although commercial splints are available, splints can be improvised using any item, or suitable material. Padded boards, tree limbs, rolled newspapers or a length of wood can each be used as a splint. An injured leg can even be splinted to the uninjured leg. In fact, any material which is the required length and wide enough to support the injured body part can be used as a splint. The splint has to be long enough to extend past the injured area to ensure the limb or entire body part is immobilised. Padding is usually placed between the splint and the natural curves of the limb such as at the elbow, knee, wrist and ankle, or where points of pressure may occur.

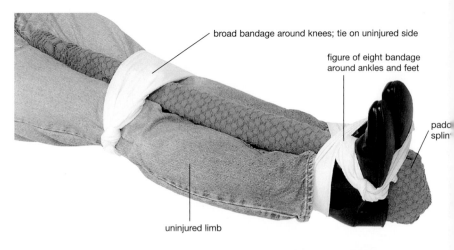

broad bandage around knees; tie on uninjured side

figure of eight bandage around ankles and feet

padd splin

uninjured limb

A broken finger or toe can best be splinted by placing gauze between it and the adjoining digit and taping them together.

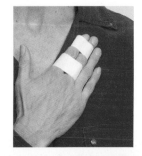

8

Safety and injury prevention

Making your environment safe will help prevent many accidents. It can save lives. Every first aider has a role to promote preventive first aid.

Remember, young children do not have a fully developed sense of danger. They are inquisitive, like to explore and are adventurous, whether in the home or outdoors. And they can be very quiet! As children cannot fully protect themselves, we as adults must do all we can to ensure a safe environment.

The precautionary measures that follow should be used as a guide for you to exercise safety and prevent injury to yourself, your family, your friends, and the community.

Remember

Keep emergency numbers and other important numbers near the telephone.

In the home

Precautions in the home are necessary to ensure the safety of everyone and to prevent injuries from occurring. When there are young children or elderly people in the home, extra precautions need to be taken.

- Make sure floors are not slippery—mop up spilt liquids and clean up grease on floors immediately.
- Don't have rugs on slippery surfaces (e.g. tiles, polished boards).
- Use ladders with care.
- Have a torch and spare batteries handy.
- Have earth leakage detectors fitted (to prevent electrocution).
- Keep a complete first aid kit.
- Check electrical cords for exposed wiring or broken covering.

Fire safety rules for the home

- Have the emergency telephone number handy—**call 000**.
- Have a fire extinguisher in a central place (not near the stove).
- Have a fire blanket or woollen blanket in the kitchen (for use on burning oil).

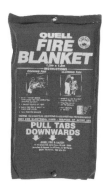

- Install smoke detectors and check regularly—change batteries annually.

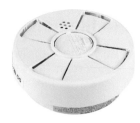

- Ensure electrical wiring and appliances are in good repair.
- Store flammable materials including matches and lighters safely.
- Be aware of the risk of falling asleep while smoking.
- Check that windows and security grilles open for an easy exit.
- Develop and practise an evacuation procedure.

In preparation in case your home is filled with smoke—teach children to **STOP DROP–ROLL** *(see p. 232)* and **GET DOWN LOW AND GO, GO, GO!**

External doors

- Keep front and back doors or at least the security doors closed.
- Make sure door knobs and latches are out of reach of young children so they cannot get out without you knowing.
- Glass doors should be made of toughened or laminated glass, with motif or decals to ensure visibility.

Hallway and stairs

- Use rugs with non-slip backing to prevent tripping and falls.
- Equip stairs with handrails.
- Ensure carpet on stairs is not loose.
- Keep halls and stairs free of toys.
- Don't let children play on public landings.
- Have stairways, corridors and dark areas well lit.

Family or lounge room

- Check for objects that may cause injury.
- Keep scissors and sewing equipment out of reach of children.
- Use dummy plugs in all unused power points.

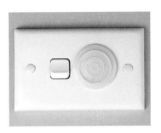

- Place trailing electrical cords out of reach of young children.
- Have eye level markings on glass doors and floor-to-ceiling windows.
- Have guards on heaters and open fireplaces.

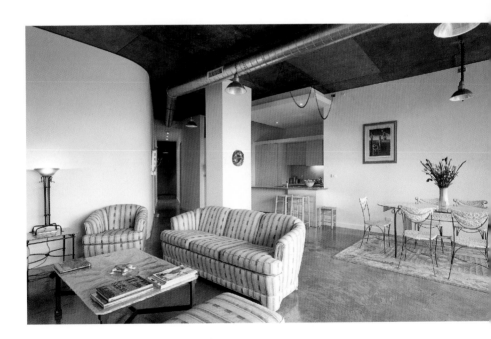

Bedroom

- Do not smoke in bed.
- Have safety rails on top bunks.
- Keep perfume, hairspray, aftershave and makeup out of reach of children.
- Don't leave a glass within reach of toddlers or crawling children.

Kitchen

- Keep out of reach of children:
  - electrical cords
  - hot food and liquids
  - knife handles
  - saucepan handles (turn them away from edge of stove).

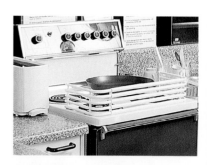

- Lift lids off hot food so that steam escapes away from you.

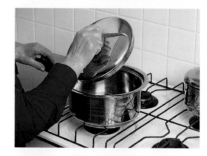

- Teach children the dangers of stoves, ovens, fireplaces, hot water taps, candles and matches.
- Use safety-designed jugs, saucepans, electrical cords, and stove guards.

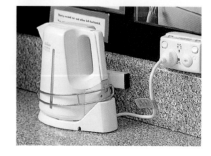

- Unplug appliances when not in use.
- Ensure electrical cords are not worn.
- Have electrical goods checked regularly for unsafe wear.

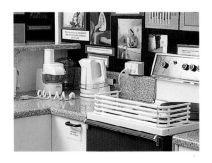

- Store domestic cleaners safely.
- Store plastic bags safely.
- Fit cupboards with childproof locks.
- Use place mats in preference to a tablecloth (small children may pull anything on a cloth onto themselves).
- Don't leave young children alone in kitchen or bathroom.
- Don't put knives and other metal objects into toasters.
- Store sharp knives safely.

Bathroom

- When preparing a bath, run cold water first, add hot water to bring to the required temperature, then finish with cold water.

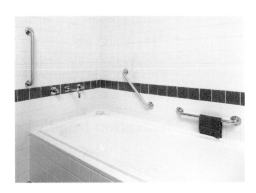

- Don't leave young children alone in bathroom or kitchen.
- Use non-slip mats in wet areas.
- Watch children in the bath.
- Don't allow electrical equipment in wet areas.
- Keep floor dry.

- Keep razor blades and shavers out of reach of children.
- Fit handrails on flights of steps and in showers and toilets.

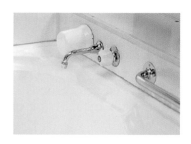

Laundry

- Store soaps, detergents and other cleaning products safely.
- Dry up spilt water.
- Have washing machines serviced regularly.
- Store poisonous substances including washing powder out of reach of children.
- Ensure that nappy bucket has a firm fitting lid and is placed off the floor.

Food

- Keep food at the correct temperature.
- Don't use food which you think may be contaminated.
- Learn and use correct hygiene principles.
- Clean preparation areas and boards with a bleach solution (1/2 tsp to 500 ml water).
- Clean cutting boards between food groups.

Medication (medicine)

- Read labels on medication carefully and take only as directed.
- Don't take someone else's medication.
- Don't take medication in front of children—they may imitate you.
- Don't dispose of unused medications in the garbage, the sink, or by flushing down the toilet.
- Take any unused or out-of-date medicines to your pharmacy for disposal.
- Teach children to recognise warning labels and poison symbols.

- Store medicines out of reach of children.
- Make sure you follow the directions on medication packets correctly.
- Make sure that medications are kept in their original container.

Babies and young children

Some extra safety precautions have to be taken when there is a baby or a young child in the house. Babies and young children do not have a fully developed sense of danger. Young children are very curious and eager to explore their environment. If there are older children, care has to be taken with some of their toys which may be dangerous for babies and young children.

- Use a safety harness in a highchair.
- Teach children not to open the door to strangers.
- Use a playpen when necessary to keep baby safe.
- Don't leave baby unattended on a change table or bed.
- Don't use a pillow for a baby in a cot; the baby could suffocate.
- Always put your baby to sleep on the back with feet at the foot of the cot—to lessen the risk of SIDS.
- Don't leave children unattended on or near stairs.
- Fit safety gate across doorways, foot of stairs or upper landing.

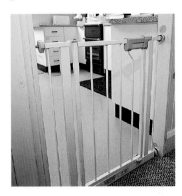

- Use a soft, level surface (e.g. woodchips) under swings and other play equipment:

  - teach children to use equipment properly.

- Only use childproof containers.
- Store chemicals out of reach of children and in a locked cupboard.
- Secure electrical cords out of reach of children.
- Turn power points off and, if there are young children, fit child proof dummy plugs.

Toys and clothing

- Clothing should be of non-flammable material.
- Clothing should be form-fitting if likely to be worn near open fires or radiators.
- Keep toys or other objects with small parts away from children (they could choke).
- Make sure toys don't have sharp edges.
- Buy non-toxic paints and crayons.
- Check warnings on the packaging of toys.
- Avoid novelty toys that are not designed to be played with by young children.

Outside the house

- Keep firm lids on garbage bins.
- Wrap broken glass with thick layers of paper before placing in bin.
- Don't leave bowls of pet food lying around.
- Avoid being outside during the hottest part of the day.
- Take frequent breaks in the shade to allow body to readjust temperature.
- Drink fluids at regular intervals when exposed to the heat of the day.

- Don't wear too many layers of clothing in hot weather; wear light coloured clothes made of natural fibres.
- Cover your body with light clothing to prevent sunburn and provide insulation from radiant heat.
- Wear a hat and sunglasses.
- Apply sunscreen regularly—at least 15+.

Swimming pool

- Install a childproof fence around pool.
- Supervise children at all times when swimming.
- Cover pool, vacuum area and enclose filter equipment.
- Have a non-slip surface around pool.
- Wear eye protection when using pool chemicals.
- Store pool chemicals safety directly after use.

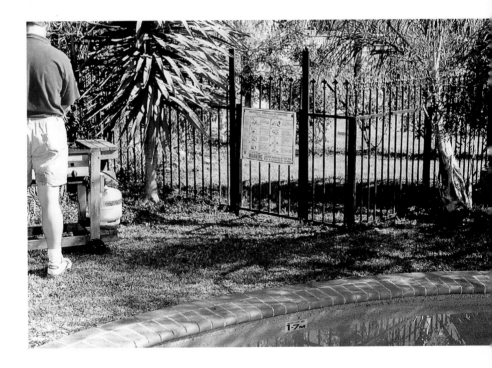

Barbecue

- Don't leave fires and lit barbecues unattended.
- Don't leave fuel and gas containers in the sun.
- Store chemicals safely and out of reach of children.
- Don't use a gas barbecue in a confined area.

Shed and garden

- Ensure backyard is fenced off from road.
- Remove doors from old refrigerators.
- Follow manufacturer's instructions when using power tools.
- Store tools safely.

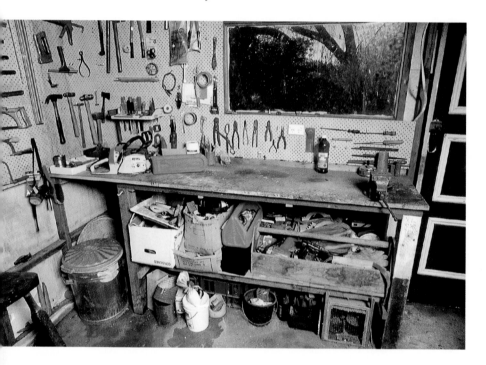

- Lock up firearms (unloaded and dismantled).
- Label and store poisons (e.g. weedkillers, kerosene) safely.
- Read safety directions before using fertilisers and poisons.

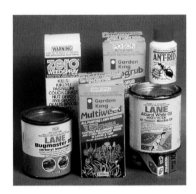

- Use eye-protection and adequate footwear when using lawnmower and other garden equipment.
- Don't put harmful products in drink or food containers.
- Ventilate areas where toxic chemicals are used—open windows and doors.
- Wear protective clothing when using chemicals.
- If spraying chemicals outside:
  - use lowest effective concentration
  - follow manufacturer's directions
  - spray when little or no wind
  - make sure no-one is in area, especially children.
- Don't dispose of unused poisonous substances by putting in garbage, emptying in sink, or flushing down toilet—return to supplier or follow directions on container.
- Turn electricity off and disconnect electrical equipment before carrying out repairs.
- Keep grass cut around house.
- When using potting mix, use protective equipment: gloves, goggles or dust mask.

Preventing insect and spider bites

- Wear insect repellent when outdoors.
- Arrange for safe removal of any nest of stinging insects near your home.
- Don't panic if a bee or wasp comes near you—teach your children not to panic.
- Wear gloves when gardening.
- Teach your children not to touch spiders.

In the workplace

- Develop and practise an emergency evacuation plan.
- Have adequate first aid supplies and be trained in their use.
- Know and follow workplace safety rules.
- If you are not sure you can lift a load or move a heavy object, don't try—get help.
- Ensure your back is straight and knees bent when lifting.
- Use warning signs to mark danger areas and dangerous equipment.
- Wear personal protective gear appropriate for the task.

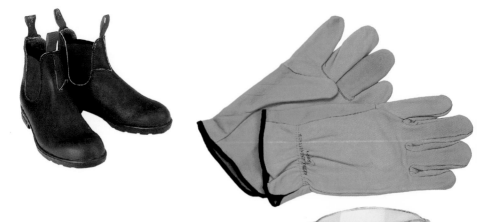

- Have fire extinguishers readily accessible.
- Keep work areas tidy.
- Ensure floors are clean and surfaces are even.
- NEVER tamper with or override safety devices on machinery.
- Ensure HAZCHEM signs are displayed when necessary.
- Wear safety belts and lifelines if working in high places.

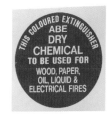

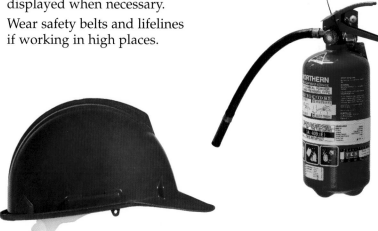

- Wear a 'hard hat' if specified for the workplace.
- Make sure any structure on which you are working is firmly secured.
- Use a tractor with caution, especially on slopes or when pulling a load.
- Mark slippery areas clearly to warn others.
- Make sure carpet is laid properly.
- Don't have rugs on slippery surfaces (e.g. tiles).
- Make sure stairs are well lit and have handrails.
- Make sure ladders are stable before use.
- Don't use chairs to stand on.

Road safety

- Hold a small child's hand when crossing the road together.
- Always cross the road at a pedestrian crossing, a corner or traffic lights, or use an underpass or overpass.

Car

- Always wear seatbelts.
- Always use age/weight appropriate safety restraints for babies and young children.
- Secure safety restraints correctly.
- Ensure car is roadworthy.
- Ensure children outside the car are in full view when you reverse the car.
- Ensure children are never left unattended in a car.
- Don't let a child play with car windows, whether manual or electric.
- Use child locks on rear doors with young children.
- Don't leave cigarettes, matches, or cigarette lighters in a car.
- Don't leave articles on rear shelf.
- Obey road signs and traffic laws.
- Don't drive if over blood alcohol limit.
- Carry a first aid kit in the car.
- Drive defensively and avoid unsafe driving practices.

Bike

- Wear bright clothes when riding a bike.
- Wear helmet when riding a bicycle or motorbike.
- Carry a first aid kit on extended bicycle rides.
- Make sure you take water to drink on long rides.

At the beach

- Swim only on patrolled beaches, between the flags.
- Obey lifesavers' instructions.
- Supervise children at all times at the beach.
- Don't swim in waters where there are warning signs.
- Use protective clothing and sunscreen (at least 15+).
- Dress young children in UV resistant clothing.
- Wear a hat and sunglasses.
- Be aware of any medications which make your skin more sensitive to the sun.

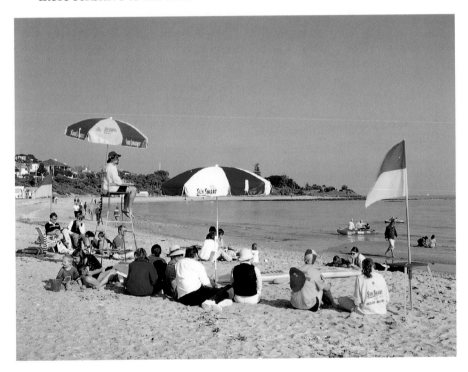

Preventing marine animal bites and stings:

- Don't step on or pick up bluebottles washed up on the sand
- Don't touch marine creatures in the water
- Wear protective shoes and wetsuit or bodystocking when necessary.

Swimming

- Avoid swimming in isolated rivers or dams unless accompanied by other people.
- Check water depth before diving into any water.
- Supervise children at all times near water.
- Don't get into a swimming hole unless there is a clear way out.
- Avoid alcohol before swimming.
- Avoid swimming in cold water for long periods.
- Don't swim in creeks and rivers known to be crocodile habitat

Water rescue

- Only attempt a water rescue if you are a strong swimmer, and the water is not too deep for you.

Boating

- Carry safety equipment and sufficient fuel and water.
- Always carry appropriate communication equipment.
- Know the distress signals and local regulations for boating.
- Ensure boat engine is in good working order before use.
- Ensure there are no petrol spills or leaks when boating.
- Always tell someone where you are going and what time you expect to be back.
- Always slow down near swimmers and small boats.
- Have sufficient lifejackets on board for everyone.
- Use protective clothing and sunscreen (at least 15+)
- Wear sunglasses and a hat.
- Only use your boat in good weather— always check weather forecast.

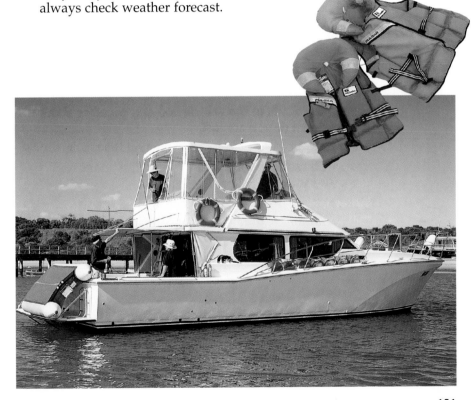

Exercising

- Warm up before exercising and don't push yourself beyond your limit.
- Remain well clear of someone swinging a bat, golf club or racquet.
- Wear a helmet for cricket, and horse riding.
- Prevent exposure to heat by:
  - avoiding strenuous exercise during hottest part of day
  - exercising in the cool of early morning of evening.
- Wear protective headgear and knee and elbow pads when skating or skateboarding.
- Don't resume exercise until fully recovered from an injury.
- Make sure there are no hazards in the exercising area which could cause a fall.

In a remote area

- Carry adequate supplies of water (at least 4 litres per person per day, stored in the shade).
- Rest in the shade of the vehicle and stay together if vehicle breaks down or you are lost.
- Wear hats, long sleeves and trousers and thick-soled boots.
- Take a CB radio, mobile phone or satellite phone for communication.
- Know how to lay adequate signals for rescuers.
- Tell authorities (e.g. rangers, police, station owners) where you are going and expected arrival times.

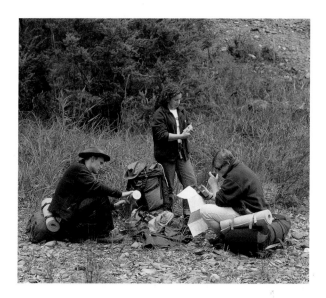

In the bush

- Always hike or camp with companions.
- Inform someone about where you are going, and when you plan to arrive and return.
- Take water, adequate food, matches, compass and map of the area.
- Take a mobile phone or portable CB radio.
- Wait for help if lost and stay with companions.
- Label all dangerous items clearly.
- Make sure stoves and lanterns are safe.
- Ensure containers of hot food cannot be tipped over.
- Ensure collapsible tables and chairs are safe.
- Protect yourself against sunburn and insect bites.
- Make sure your camp fire is out before leaving.
- Know how to prevent and treat overexposure to heat or cold.
- Wear appropriate clothes and thick-soled shoes.

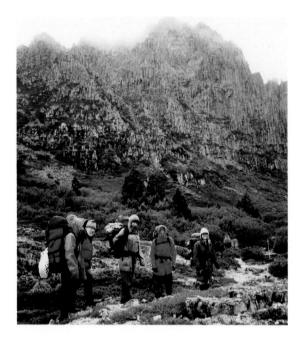

- Carry an appropriate first aid kit.
- When camping, store food and drink out of reach of animals.
- Don't feed wild animals.

To avoid tick bites:

- wear a long-sleeved shirt with a firm collar and cuffs and tuck pants into socks or boots when walking through the bush or long grass
- check your body for ticks after walking in the bush.

To avoid snakebite:

- make a lot of noise when walking in the bush
- always wear shoes outside
- be aware of snakes' habits.

  Do not:
  - put hands or feet where you cannot see what is there
  - put your hand into a hollow log

- reach into long grass
- pick up a 'stick' unless you have checked it carefully.

• If climbing, don't reach up and put your hand on a ledge or rock without checking first.

• Teach children to keep clear of snakes.

• Be extremely wary of all snakes—keep away!

What to do in the case of fire

Evacuating from a burning building

Fires can burn and spread very quickly in a building—even a minor fire can escalate in minutes to a serious blaze. Often smoke and fumes from the fire are more dangerous than the flames. It is easy to be overcome by smoke and a lack of oxygen. Furnishings containing synthetic materials give off toxic fumes when burning.

Panic is another danger which can spread very quickly. Therefore, it is important to remain calm and to calm anyone else involved.

Home or building on fire

1 Remain calm.

2 **Call 000** for emergency services—from a place outside building, if necessary.

3 Activate any fire alarms.

4 Extinguish the fire, if possible.

If it becomes necessary to leave the building:

5 Shut doors and windows to contain fire.

6 Carry out evacuation procedure.

7 Leave the building quickly without running.

8 Turn power off, if possible.

9 DO NOT go back inside for anything.

8

A fire in a large building (e.g. hotel, office block) can be extremely dangerous and knowing how to get out could mean the difference between life and death. When you first go into an unfamiliar building, check where the fire exits and the fire extinguishers are located. If you have to be evacuated, follow the instructions of those organising the evacuation.

Fire in a large building—additional points

1 DO NOT use lifts under any circumstances.

2 DO NOT open a door if it feels hot.

3 If unable to get to fire exit, return to your room/office:

- push wet towels and cloths into any cracks (e.g. under doors and windows) and vents

- turn off ventilation system (if possible)

- call the front desk or emergency services to report the fire and your location.

4 DO NOT enter a burning building—leave it to emergency services.

5 If overhead high voltage lines are involved, wait for electricity authorities and direct others away.

6 If casualties are affected by any of the following, move them to fresh air:

- asphyxia (lack of oxygen)

- carbon monoxide poisoning

- poisoning from toxic fumes

- irritation of respiratory tract and eyes.

Bushfires

In Australia those who live in rural areas or in a city, are at risk of exposure to bushfires. There are a number of long-term measures you can take to protect your home.

Remember

Anyone in or near bushfire-prone areas should familiarise themselves with local guidelines and recommendations.

- Clear a fuel break of about 30–40 metres around the home.
- Make sure gutters are clear of leaves and other vegetation.
- Clear undergrowth, overhanging branches and any flammable material and liquids from around the house.
- Fit windows, vents, chimneys and doors with screens to stop sparks from entering.
- Seal off area under house.
- Ensure access to your own emergency water supply (there may be no mains pressure during a fire).
- Prepare a fire evacuation plan—late evacuation is a very dangerous option.
- Prepare an emergency kit to include heavy cotton clothing, long-sleeved top and long trousers, leather shoes and gloves, face covering, torches, bottles of water and battery operated radio.

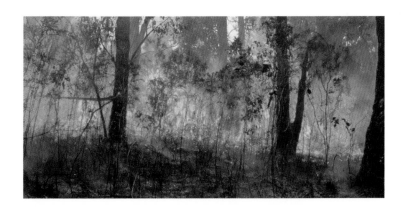

When a bushfire is in the vicinity of your home, there are further measures you can take.

- Put on clothing from emergency kit.
- Carry out your plan; if evacuating LEAVE EARLY and take pets.
- Plug downpipes with sand or earth-filled bags.
- Fill gutters with water.
- Hose those parts of the building where fire could take hold.
- Dampen the ground around the house.
- Put wet, rolled towels under doors and around windows.
- Close windows.
- Place furniture away from windows.
- Secure pets in house if you haven't evacuated.

Note: *Wet towels and woollen or cotton blankets can be used for personal protection against fire and to minimise smoke inhalation.*

Wounds and bleeding

The skin

The skin is the body's largest organ. It plays an important role in protecting the body from infection and performs a number of other important functions. The skin:

- acts as a shield against injury
- when intact, protects internal organs against invasion by environmental microbes
- is waterproof and helps regulate the body's temperature
- alerts the brain to changes in the environment (from receptors of the skin).

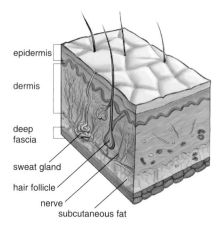

The outer layer or epidermis acts as a barrier to bacteria and other organisms that cause infection. A deeper layer, called the dermis, contains the main nerve structures, sweat and oil glands and blood vessels. There are an abundance of nerves in the skin. These are sensitive to touch, heat, cold and pain, and transmit these sensations to the brain. Because the skin has a plentiful supply of nerves and blood vessels, most superficial injuries are likely to bleed and be painful.

Bleeding

Blood is vital for the body to function properly and has many important functions—transporting oxygen and nutrients to all parts of the body, eliminating wastes, transporting antibodies to protect against disease and germs, and maintaining a constant body temperature.

Bleeding is the loss of blood from the blood vessels. This can be external and obvious, or internal (within the body) where it often cannot be seen. When there is an open wound and blood loss, the bleeding must be stopped and the possibility of infection and shock has to be considered, whether the wound is major or minor.

Bleeding is classified according to the type of blood vessel that is damaged—artery, vein or capillary.

Arterial blood is oxygen-rich, bright red in colour and under pressure, so it spurts (sometimes pulsing) from the wound. Because this makes it more difficult for the blood to clot, arterial bleeding is hardest to control.

Venous blood (from the veins) is oxygen-depleted, dark red in colour and under less pressure. It flows from a wound more evenly and without spurting.

Capillary bleeding (bright red in colour) is the most common form of bleeding and is usually slow because the blood vessels are small and under low pressure. Clotting occurs easily with this type of bleeding. If capillaries are ruptured beneath the skin's surface, blood escapes into the surrounding tissues and bruising results.

Whether the bleeding is external or internal, it is important for the first aider to know from other signs and symptoms how serious the blood loss is. Some wounds may be minor but can still cause pain and, if not managed correctly, may become more serious later.

SIGNS AND SYMPTOMS OF MAJOR BLEEDING

- faintness or dizziness
- restlessness
- nausea
- thirst
- weak, rapid pulse
- cold, clammy skin
- rapid, gasping breathing
- pallor
- sweating
- progressive loss of consciousness (drowsy, irrational or unconscious).

Internal bleeding poses special challenges to the first aider and has to be recognised and treated with care. It can be difficult to assess how serious internal bleeding is. Some wounds are life-threatening and need urgent attention.

SIGNS AND SYMPTOMS OF INTERNAL BLEEDING

- pain
- tenderness
- rigidity of abdominal muscles
- other signs of blood loss *(see p. 217)*.

Aims in managing bleeding

Ensure your hands are clean and gloved— whenever possible.

1   Control bleeding.

2   Apply pressure to the wound to restrict the flow of blood and allow normal clotting to occur (use a pad and dressing).

3   Raise the injured part to slow the flow of blood and encourage clotting.

4   Maintain pressure on the pad (by hand, or by the use a triangular or roller bandage).

5 Minimise shock—this may result from extensive
loss of blood, emotional distress or pain.

6 Minimise the risk of infection—cover wound with
a sterile bandage (if available).

7 Consider the need for medical aid.

Major external bleeding requires rapid medical attention.
Remember, where there is extensive blood loss, it can distract
from the priorities of resuscitation. Rarely is blood loss so
great that the heart stops.

Checking circulation (blood supply)

If the bleeding is on the limb, the supply of blood in the hand
or foot must be checked regularly after any bandage, splint
or sling has been applied. This is important as swelling of the
limb can make the bandage tighter. If circulation is impaired
the bandage must be loosened.

SIGNS AND SYMPTOMS OF A BANDAGE BEING TOO TIGHT

- absent pulse below the bandage
- swelling
- paleness, blueness or coldness of the fingers or toes
- numbness and tingling (pins and needles)
of the fingers or toes
- pain.

HOW TO CHECK CIRCULATION (BLOOD SUPPLY)

- Check skin colour—if not normal, blood supply
could be impaired.
- Check skin temperature—if cold, blood supply could
be impaired.
- Check for blood supply in fingers or toes by pressing
fingernail or toenail until it turns white, then release—if
colour returns within 2 seconds, blood supply is
unrestricted.

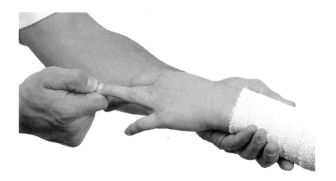

Note: *If nail is already blue or white or numb, loosen bandage.*

Infection and wounds

Open wounds may become infected as a result of micro-organisms entering the wound from the skin or the air; or from germs on the object which caused the wound. Wounds are also likely to become infected if any foreign matter, dead tissue or bacteria remain in the wound.

If the first aider's skin is not intact (open wound, dermatitis, laceration or ulcer), germs from the casualty's body fluids may enter into the first aider's body. The first aider should always have their own non-intact skin covered and use disposable gloves whenever possible.

It is possible that the first aider's skin may be penetrated accidentally by a needle contaminated with the casualty's blood or body fluid. Regardless of the infectious status of the casualty, anyone who receives a 'needle-stick' injury needs special care, management and follow up *(for the management of a needle-stick injury see p. 137).*

A wound that has not begun to heal within two days may be infected. Infections can spread through the body and become life-threatening.

SIGNS OF INFECTION

- increased pain and soreness
- increased temperature (warmth) around wound area
- increased swelling and redness of the wound and surrounding area
- pus oozing from the wound
- fever (if the infection persists)
- swelling and tenderness of the lymph glands
- tracking or red streak leading away from the wound.

Management of infected wounds

1 Clean and dress wound with sterile dressing and bandage.

2 Elevate, if a limb, and immobilise.

3 Seek medical attention.

Tetanus

Tetanus is a potentially fatal disease caused by infection with the tetanus bacterium. The bacteria enter through an open wound or burn and bacterial toxins affect the body's nervous system.

SIGNS AND SYMPTOMS

- stiffness of the jaw (lockjaw, often the first sign)
- difficulty swallowing
- a stiff neck
- irritability and headaches
- chills and fever
- generalised stiffness
- spasms—local or general.

Tetanus immunisation lasts for many years if the childhood/adolescent schedule of vaccination is adhered to. Ordinarily, a booster is not required until a person reaches 50 years of age **or** if they sustain a tetanus-prone wound. Whenever any casualty sustains a wound ask if tetanus immunisation is current. If not, casualty should seek medical advice.

Tetanus-prone wounds

Types of wounds likely to favour the growth of tetanus organisms include compound fractures, deep penetrating wounds, wounds containing foreign bodies (especially wood splinters), wounds with extensive tissue damage (e.g. contusion or burn), and any superficial wound obviously contaminated with soil, dust or horse manure (especially if disinfection is delayed more than four hours). Replacement, of an avulsed (knocked-out) tooth is also a tenanus-prone event, as minimal washing and cleaning of the tooth is conducted to increase the likelihood of successful replacement.

External bleeding

External bleeding occurs most often after a deep cut (incision) or tear (laceration) in the skin. Most severe bleeding usually occurs from arteries, although varicose veins (most commonly found in the legs) can also bleed heavily *(see p. 214)*.

Management of external bleeding

1 Follow **DRABCD**.

2 Lie casualty down if bleeding is severe.

3 Remove or cut clothing to expose the wound.

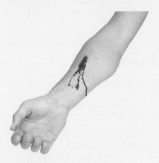

4 Apply firm direct pressure—instruct casualty to do this if possible.

5 If casualty is unable to apply pressure, apply pressure using a pad or your hands (use gloves if available).

6 Squeeze the wound edges together if possible.

7 Elevate the bleeding part— restrict movement as much as possible.

8 Apply a pad over the wound if not already in place and secure with bandage—ensure pad remains over wound.

9 If bleeding still not controlled, leave initial pad in place and apply a second pad—secure with a bandage.

10 If bleeding continues through second pad, replace the second pad (only) and bandage.

11 If bleeding is severe or persistent, give nothing by mouth—**call 000** for an ambulance.

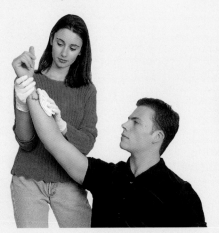

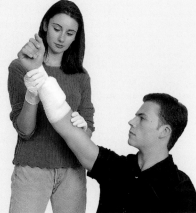

Constrictive bandage

Occasionally, in major limb injuries such as partial amputations or large crater wounds (e.g. shark attack), severe bleeding cannot be controlled by direct pressure. In this situation only, it may be necessary as a last resort to apply a constrictive bandage above the elbow or knee to restrict arterial blood flow. Care must be taken as its prolonged use can lead to tissues being starved of blood and dying.

Applying a constrictive bandage

1   Use a firm cloth, at least 5 cm wide and about 75 cm long (improvise with clothing or a folded triangular bandage).

2   Wrap the cloth strip firmly around the injured limb—between elbow and shoulder, or knee and pelvis—until a pulse can no longer be felt beyond the constrictive bandage and bleeding has been controlled.

3   Note the time of application; write this on the casualty in pen.

4   **Call 000** for an ambulance.

5   After 30 minutes, release the bandage and check for bleeding:

   • if there is no bleeding, remove the constrictive bandage

   • if bleeding recommences, apply direct pressure

   • if direct pressure is unsuccessful, reapply constrictive bandage; recheck every 30 minutes.

Ensure bandage is clearly visible and a written tag is on the casualty. Inform medical aid (ambulance) of the position of bandage and time of application.

Note: In the rare case where a constrictive bandage is required; if it is applied too loosely, the bleeding can be made worse. It must stop the arterial pulse below the bandage..

Open wounds

An open wound is where there is a break in the outer layer of skin. Open wounds may be minor (e.g. a surface scrape) or more severe (e.g. when an object penetrates deeply to underlying layers). Remember, there may be a broken bone under an open wound. Although the amount of bleeding will depend on how bad the injury is, any open wound provides a gateway for germs to enter the body and cause infection.

Note: Dirty, penetrating, or open wounds should be examined by a doctor, as tetanus or other serious infections may result especially if there is dirt or foreign material in the wound.

Infection transmission to you and the casualty can be minimised by:

- washing and drying your hands thoroughly before and after giving first aid, even if you are wearing gloves
- wearing clean disposable gloves, whether there is or is not a likelihood of exposure to blood or body fluid
- avoiding coughing, sneezing or talking while managing the wound
- handling the wound only when it is necessary to control severe bleeding
- using sterile or clean dressings.

The general principles for applying dressings are:

- wash and dry hands before you put on clean disposable gloves
- use a sterile dressing that extends about 2 cm past the edges of the wound
- do not touch the dressing surface that will contact the wound
- if the wound is minor, clean with sterile saline or clean water (if not available, use an antiseptic swab) before applying a dressing.
- replace at least once a day any dressing which becomes wet or soiled with blood or pus at least once a day
- wash and dry hands after removing gloves.

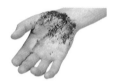 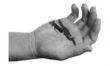

	Bruise (Contusion)	Abrasion	Cut (Incision)
Kind of wound	closed	open	open
Caused by	blow from something blunt	skin being scraped across a hard surface	something sharp (e.g. knife or glass)
Injury causes	vessels under skin to bleed into surrounding tissues	outer layer of skin and tiny underlying blood vessels to be exposed	skin, soft tissue or muscles to be severed
Management	• RICE *(see p. 159)*	• clean wound • apply non-adherent dressing	• clean wound thoroughly with sterile gauze soaked in saline (if available) or in cooled, boiled water • apply non-adherent dressing

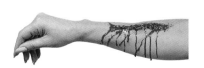

	Laceration	Puncture	Tear (Avulsion)
Kind of wound	open	open	open
Caused by	machinery, barbed wire, teeth or claws	blunt or pointed instruments	severe force
Injury causes	skin and underlying tissue damage	skin and underlying tissue damage and possibly infection	skin and other soft tissues to be partially or completely torn away
Management	• clean wound thoroughly with sterile gauze soaked in saline (if available), or in cooled, boiled water • apply non-adherent dressing	• clean wound thoroughly with sterile gauze soaked in saline (if available), or in cooled, boiled water • apply non-adherent dressing	• return skin to original position if possible • apply pressure to wound using a a pad, with hand pressure of a dressing to control any bleeding • bandage

9

Major wounds

Embedded object

When a foreign object such as a knife, glass, branch or stick is embedded in the wound and has penetrated into tissue:

- **DO NOT** try to remove the object as it may be plugging the wound and restricting bleeding. Removing it may result in severe bleeding or may damage deep structures.

- **DO NOT** exert any pressure over the object.

- **DO NOT** try to cut the end of the object unless its size makes it unmanageable.

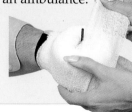

Management of embedded object

1 Control bleeding by applying pressure to the surrounding areas but not on the foreign object.

2 Place padding around the object or place a ring pad over the object and a bandage over the padding.

3 If the length of the object causes it to protrude outside the pad, take care to bandage only each side of the object.

4 Seek medical aid or consider calling 000 for an ambulance.

Puncture wounds

Puncture wounds are serious and may occur when a knife, or high velocity object such as a bullet, has penetrated the skin. The penetration may be deep and infection will occur. There may be a wound where the object has left the body and this must also be treated.

Management of puncture wounds

1 Control bleeding—apply direct pressure around the wound.

2 Keep wound as clean as possible.

3 Cut away or remove clothing covering the wound.

4 If wound is not bleeding, carefully clean around the wound.

5 DO NOT try to pick out foreign material embedded in the wound. Also check for an exit wound from a puncture wound.

6 Apply a sterile or clean dressing.

7 Rest the injured part in a comfortable position.

8 Seek medical aid—consider calling 000 for an ambulance.

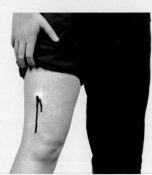

Blast injuries

Blast injuries can result from an explosion in the workplace (e.g. from explosives or chemicals), at home (e.g. from a gas heater), from fireworks or as a result of terrorist attack. The casualty may be injured because of being thrown by the blast, struck by material thrown by the blast, or may suffer injuries to the lungs, stomach or intestines, or loss of hearing caused by shock waves from the blast.

SIGNS AND SYMPTOMS

- coughing up frothy blood
- chest pain
- possible bleeding from ears
- possible fractures
- multiple soft tissue injuries
- shock.

Management of blast injuries

1 Follow **DRABCD**.

2 **Call 000** for an ambulance.

3 Place casualty in comfortable position.

4 Control bleeding.

5 Care for wounds and burns.

6 Immobilise any fractures.

7 Monitor breathing and other vital signs.

Amputated parts

An amputation occurs when a part of the body such as a toe, finger, hand, or leg is partly or completely cut off, or is torn off. The first aider aims to:

- minimise blood loss and shock
- preserve the amputated part because it may be possible to re-attach a finger or limb by microsurgery; the first aider will need to care for the amputated part in addition to the casualty.

Management of amputations

The casualty

1 Follow **DRABCD**.

2 **Call 000** for an ambulance.

3 Apply direct pressure to the wound and raise the limb to control blood loss.

4 Apply a sterile dressing and bandage.

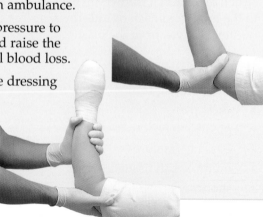

The amputated part

1   DO NOT wash or soak the amputated part in water or any other liquid.

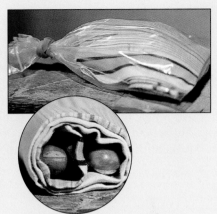

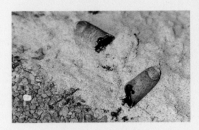

2   Wrap the part in gauze or material and place in a watertight container, such as a sealed watertight plastic bag.

3   Place the sealed container in cold water which has had ice added to it (if available). The severed part should not be in direct contact with ice.

4   Send to hospital with the casualty.

Wounds to head and face

Bleeding from the scalp

The head is easily injured because it lacks the padding of other parts of the body. An injury to this part of the body is of particular concern because of the possibility of injury to the skull.

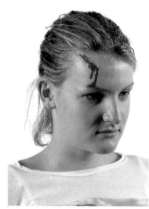

Management of bleeding from the scalp

1   Follow **DRABCD**.

2   If you suspect a fracture, control bleeding with gentle pressure around the wound.

3   If there appears to be no fracture, control bleeding with firm, direct pressure (wear gloves; use a pad if available and bandage).

4   If the casualty's general condition and other injuries permit, sitting up may help reduce bleeding.

5   Monitor the casualty's condition.

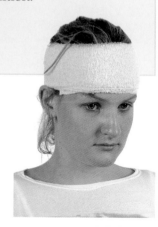

Ear wounds

Ear injuries are common. Sport injuries and falls can damage the outer soft tissue, causing a bleed. Bleeding can be controlled by applying pressure to the affected area.

A direct blow to the head or pushing something into the ear may result in internal injury to the eardrum.

Management of bleeding from within the ear

1 Follow **DRABCD**.

2 DO NOT plug ear canal.

3 DO NOT administer drops of any kind.

4 Allow fluid to drain freely.

5 Place casualty on side with affected ear down.

6 Place a sterile pad between ear and the ground.

7 **Call 000** for an ambulance.

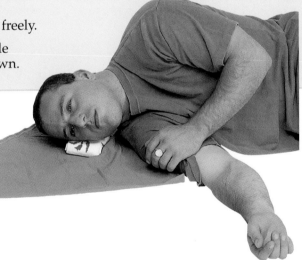

Foreign objects in the ear

Foreign objects such as beads, stones and grass seeds can become lodged in the canal. If an insect flies or crawls into the ear, it is always quite alarming. The insect can usually be floated out with warmed vegetable oil (e.g. olive oil) or water.

Management of a foreign object in the ear

Foreign object in ear

1 Look in the ear to identify the object and to see how deeply it is lodged.

2 DO NOT attempt to remove object.

3 Seek medical aid.

Small insect in ear

1 Gently pour some vegetable oil (water if oil not available), warmed to body temperature, into the ear canal.

2 If insect does not float out, seek medical aid.

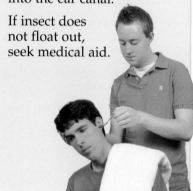

Dental injuries and wounds

Bleeding may result from a blow to the mouth which knocks teeth out, or may follow a tooth extraction or a loose tooth. The most important action is to ensure the casualty maintains a clear airway.

If an adult tooth is knocked out, it may be replaced in the socket. If you are unable to place it back in the socket, store it in casualty's own saliva or milk. If these are not available, use sterile saline until dental attention is available.

If the knocked-out tooth is from a child under seven years (primary tooth/baby), do not attempt to replace the tooth as there is a risk of damaging the underlying permanent tooth. A dentist should check the child's gum. Try to find the tooth to ensure it has not been swallowed.

Management of dental injuries and wounds

1 Maintain a clear airway.

2 Instruct the casualty to keep their tongue clear of tooth socket.

3 Place firm pad of gauze over socket.

4 Instruct the casualty to bite firmly on gauze.

5 If bleeding continues, seek medical or dental aid.

Replacing an adult knocked-out tooth

1 Gently clean dirt off tooth with casualty's own saliva or milk. If not available, use sterile saline solution. Failing these, use clean tap water.

2 Put tooth back in the open socket—unless casualty is a child under seven years (primary/baby tooth).

3 Ask the casualty to hold tooth in place. If unable to replace, wrap tooth in plastic or store in milk or sterile saline and rush casualty and tooth to a dentist.

4 If tooth has been in contact with dirt or soil, advise having a tetanus injection.

5 Advise the casualty to see a dentist as soon as possible.

Note: This management also applies to children over seven years who have permanent (adult) teeth.

Nosebleeds

Nosebleeds can have various causes such as a blow to the nose, excessive blowing, sneezing, high blood pressure and changes in altitude. Many nosebleeds have no obvious cause.

Management of nosebleeds

1 Ask the casualty to breathe through mouth and not to blow nose.

2 Sit the casualty up, head slightly forward.

3 Apply finger and thumb pressure on soft part of nostrils below bridge of nose for at least 10 minutes.

4 Loosen tight clothing around neck.

5 Place cold wet towels (or ice wrapped in a wet cloth) on the neck and forehead.

6 If bleeding persists, seek medical aid.

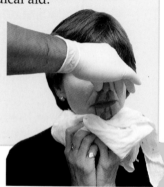

Other wounds and bleeding

Bleeding from the palm

Bleeding from the palm may be severe as several blood vessels can be involved. There may also be damage to bones and nerves.

Management of bleeding from palm of hand

1   If there is no object embedded, apply firm direct pressure to palm using a pad or something similar.

2   Bandage hand and fingers firmly using a triangular or broad roller bandage.

3   Elevate hand in St John sling.

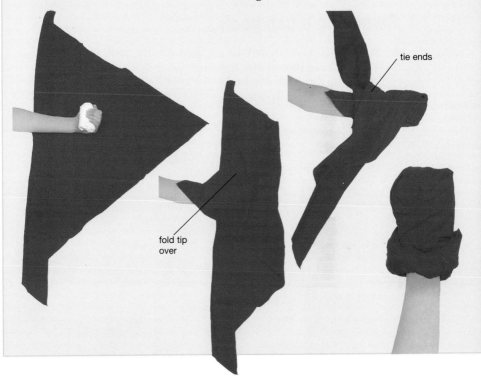

tie ends

fold tip over

To contain the bleeding and to apply pressure to the palm, you can use:

- a triangular bandage
- an unopened roller bandage
- a clean cloth wrapped around an object such as a matchbox or smooth stone
- two or three fingers of the undamaged hand.

A St John sling will elevate the hand to control the bleeding.

Fish hook wounds

If medical aid is not readily available and the hook is embedded just under the skin, attempt to remove it using the steps below—but only make the one attempt. If you are unsuccessful, manage as for an embedded object (see p. 202).

Removing a fish hook

1   If the barb is embedded, loop fishing line along curve or throat of the hook and grip firmly in one hand.

2   Press down on the shank of the hook with thumb of other hand.

3   Pull the hook straight out.

4   If the barb is protruding, cut it off and withdraw the hook.

5   Seek medical aid.

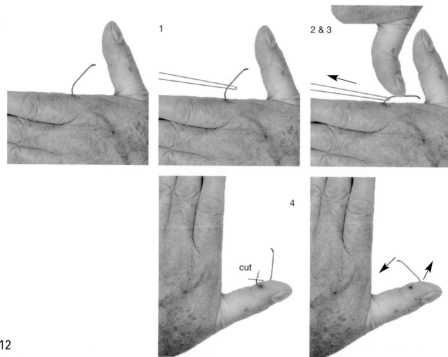

Splinter removal

Superficial splinters—where the splinter end protrudes from the skin or is visible under the surface of the skin—may be removed using the steps below.

Removing a splinter

1   Put on protective gloves to minimise infection.

2   Clean the area around the splinter with soap and water.

3   If the splinter end protrudes from the skin, grasp the splinter with cleaned tweezers and pull the splinter out at the angle it went in.

4   If the splinter end is not protruding from the skin, expose the splinter using a disposable sterile splinter probe, then remove it as in Step 3.

5   Clean the area with an antiseptic swab and apply a transparent or adhesive dressing.

6   Seek medical advice if:

   • splinter area becomes more painful, reddened and swollen

   or

   • splinter breaks or does not come out easily.

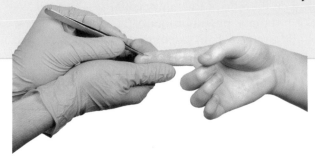

Bleeding from varicose veins

The veins in the legs contain valves to keep the blood flowing towards the heart. When the valves deteriorate, blood leaks backwards and the pressure from the blood causes the vein to become swollen and knotted ('varicose'). They may bleed profusely if injured.

Management of bleeding varicose veins

1 Apply a clean pad and bandage firmly.

2 Place the casualty flat with legs raised.

3 Remove any constricting items from limb.

4 Seek medical aid.

Penetrating chest wound

A penetrating chest wound can cause severe internal damage within both the chest and upper abdomen. The lungs are particularly vulnerable to injury. If a puncture is deep enough, the rib cage may be penetrated allowing air to enter the chest through the wound. When air enters this space (pleural cavity), the lung on the side of the injury collapses. This is called an open or traumatic pneumothorax. Pressure in the chest cavity may build up to such an extent that the heart is pushed to the side. Thus the function of the uninjured lung on that side may also be affected. The build-up of pressure may also prevent adequate refilling of the heart, impairing the blood supply and causing shock.

SIGNS AND SYMPTOMS

- pain at site of wound
- unconsciousness
- difficult and painful breathing
- bloodstained bubbles around wound when casualty exhales
- sound of air being sucked into chest as the casualty inhales.

The first priority is to seal wound while allowing fluid and air to escape from wound, monitor breathing and **call 000** for an ambulance.

Management of a penetrating chest wound

1 Follow **DRABCD**.

2 Place casualty in a sitting position with affected side down.

3 Cover the wound—use the casualty's or your own hand to stop air flowing in and out of chest cavity.

4 Cover wound with a dressing such as plastic sheet, bag or aluminium foil—if not available, use a sterile dressing or pad.

5 Seal with tape on three sides (not bottom).

6 **Call 000** for an ambulance.

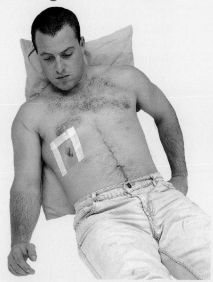

Note: Check for an exit wound, especially if caused by a velocity trauma (e.g. gunshot wound).

Vaginal bleeding

If a woman is bleeding from the vagina, it is most likely to be
associated with a monthly menstrual period. Ask the casualty
if the bleeding is associated with her periods. Ask if she is
pregnant. Vaginal bleeding in pregnancy is always serious.

Management of vaginal bleeding

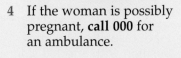

1 Take the woman to
   a private place.

2 Give her a sanitary
   pad or clean towel.

3 Make her comfortable with
   head and shoulders raised
   and supported, knees
   propped up.

4 If the woman is possibly
   pregnant, **call 000** for
   an ambulance.

*Note: If sexual assault has occurred or is suspected, follow steps
1 to 3. Seek medical and police aid urgently. Stay with the casualty.
Do not disturb evidence by removing, washing or disposing of
clothing. If possible, persuade casualty not to go to toilet until
a forensic examination has been carried out by a doctor.*

Internal bleeding

Internal bleeding occurs when blood escapes from arteries,
veins or capillaries into tissues or cavities in the body.
Although capillary bleeding (indicated by mild bruising)
is not serious, deeper bleeding involving veins and arteries
may result in severe blood loss.

Severe internal bleeding usually results from injuries caused
by a violent blunt force (such as in a car accident or fall from
a height). It can also occur when an object (e.g. a knife)
penetrates the skin and damages internal structures. Some
conditions (such as a stomach ulcer or complications of
pregnancy) can also result in internal bleeding.

Internal bleeding is usually more serious than external
bleeding. Although there is no external loss of blood, blood
is lost from the circulatory system and vital organs which may
result in shock. Internal bleeding can also cause problems if
it causes pressure on vital parts of the body such as the brain.

SIGNS AND SYMPTOMS

- pain
- tenderness
- rigidity of abdominal muscles
- distension or swelling
- other signs of blood loss, especially pallor, sweating,
  faintness or thirst.

Evidence of internal bleeding from some organs may
be seen by the first aider; for example:

- coughing up red, frothy blood
- vomiting material which is obviously blood or may
  look like coffee grounds (coloured black)
- passing faeces with a black, tarry appearance
- passing faeces which are red in colour
- passing urine which has a red or smoky appearance.

Internal bleeding may be accompanied by any of the signs
and symptoms of major bleeding. Cardiac arrest can occur if
enough blood is lost.

Management of internal bleeding

1 Lie the casualty down—a pillow may be used under the head to increase comfort.

2 If the casualty is coughing up frothy blood, allow them to adopt a position of comfort (normally half-sitting).

3 Raise the legs or bend the knees.

4 Loosen tight clothing.

5 **Call 000** for an ambulance.

6 Give nothing by mouth.

7 Calm the casualty.

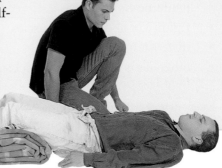

Abdominal injuries

Organs in the abdomen can easily be injured because there is no bone structure to protect them. Some of these—liver, spleen and stomach—tend to bleed easily and profusely, so injuries to them can be life-threatening. Injury to the bowel may result in the contents being spilled into the abdominal cavity, causing infection.

An injury to the abdomen can be open or closed. Both are serious as even in a closed wound an organ can be ruptured, causing serious internal bleeding and shock. With an open injury, abdominal organs can protrude through the wound.

SIGNS AND SYMPTOMS

- severe pain
- nausea or vomiting
- bruising and tenderness around the wound
- unnatural paleness
- external bleeding
- blood in the urine
- distension/swelling
- protrusion of intestines through an abdominal wound
- shock.

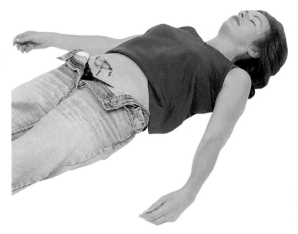

Management of abdominal injuries

1 Follow **DRABCD**.

2 Place casualty on back with knees slightly raised and supported—a pillow may be used under the head to increase comfort.

3 Loosen clothing.

4 Cover protruding organs with aluminium foil or plastic food wrap, or a large, non-stick, sterile dressing, soaked in sterile saline (clean water if saline is not available).

5 Secure with broad bandage (not tightly).

6 **Call 000** for an ambulance.

- DO NOT give anything to drink.

- DO NOT try to push organs back into abdomen.

- DO NOT apply direct pressure to the wound.

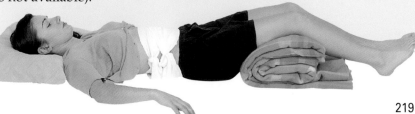

Crush injuries

A crush injury results when something large and heavy strikes or falls on a person. There are a number of situations in which this may occur, for example at a traffic accident, on a building site, at a train crash, in an explosion, during an earthquake or in a mining accident.

Crush injuries are often very serious, because the damage may cause:

- internal bleeding
- fractured bones
- ruptured organs
- impaired blood supply.

If the casualty is trapped for any length of time, there is the risk of complications such as extensive tissue damage and shock, as well as the release of toxic substances into the circulation which may lead later to acute kidney failure. This takes a number of hours to build up, therefore the urgent removal of the object is a priority. After calling for an ambulance the first aider should do whatever else is possible for the casualty.

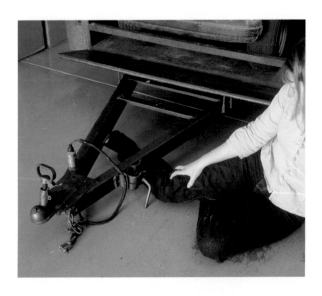

Management of crush injuries

1 Follow **DRABCD**.

2 **Call 000** for an ambulance.

3 Ensure your own safety.

4 If safe, remove the crushing object as soon as possible.

5 Control bleeding.

6 Manage other injuries.

7 Comfort and reassure the casualty.

Haematomas

A haematoma is caused by a sharp, blunt blow which does not break the skin but causes internal damage to blood vessels. This results in the accumulation of a quantity of blood at the site.

SIGNS AND SYMPTOMS

- severe pain
- area turning dark blue or red
- rapid and severe swelling
- loss of mobility of the area.

A haematoma can be quite dangerous as it may conceal underlying injuries.

Management of a haematoma

1 Follow **DRABCD**.

2 Apply RICE management:

- **rest** the casualty and the injured part

- apply **icepacks** (cold compress) wrapped in a wet cloth to the injury for 15 minutes every 2 hours for 24 hours, then for 15 minutes every 4 hours for 24 hours

- apply a **compression** bandage such as an elastic bandage firmly to extend well beyond the injury

- **elevate** the injured part.

3 Seek medical aid.

Bruise (contusion)

A bruise is an injury caused by the rupture of small blood vessels under the skin. It is an injury that does not break the skin surface. It is usually caused by a blow or a knock to the body which causes discolouration to the outer skin and is accompanied by swelling and pain. Bruising may appear rapidly if bleeding is near the surface of the skin. By immediately applying pressure and a cold compress, the extent of the bruising may be reduced.

Commonly, the bruise is accompanied by a lump which may develop within minutes after the blow or fall. In this case, treat as for a bruise but apply continual firm pressure for several minutes.

Management of a bruise (contusion)

1 Apply **RICE** management:

- **Rest** the casualty and the injured part.

- Apply **I**cepack (cold compress) wrapped in a wet cloth for 15 minutes every 2 hours for 24 hours, then for 15 minutes every 4 hours for 24 hours (if necessary).

- Apply a **C**ompression bandage firmly to extend well beyond the injury.

- **E**levate the injured part.

2 Seek medical aid if the pain is not relieved by cold compresses.

10

Burns and scalds

Burn injuries are extremely painful. Risk of infection is high because the outer layer of skin is damaged. Although they do not bleed, burn injuries result in fluid loss, loss of temperature control and can damage underlying layers of tissue and nerves. If sustained in a confined space, burns may damage the respiratory system and eyes. The casualty may go into shock as a result of fluid loss.

As well as the obvious physical damage, burns cause psychological damage as they can be disfiguring and disabling with an altered body image.

Burns are primarily caused by scalding from hot liquid or flames and contact with hot objects, but can also be caused by extreme cold, chemicals, electricity, or the sun and other forms of radiation. Even after the source of heat has been removed, further damage occurs because soft tissue retains heat for minutes afterwards.

Cooling the burnt area and preventing infection are the first aider's major objectives. In some cases, the first aider will also have to monitor the casualty and treat for respiratory distress, cardiac arrest, or shock.

Burns and scalds

Burns are injuries to the skin and underlying tissues caused by heat, extreme cold, chemicals, corrosive substances, electricity, friction such as rope burn and radiation such as the sun, microwaves, snow, sun lamps and therapeutic radiotherapy. Scalds are burns caused by hot liquid and steam.

Children under 5 are more at risk due to their smaller fluid resolve and the elderly due to associated illnesses (i.e. diabetes, respiratory or cardiac problems) and age-related degenerative changes.

The severity of a burn

The severity of a burn depends on:
- extent of burn (surface area damage)
- part(s) of body burnt, especially airway damage
- depth of burn
- age and physical condition of casualty
- associated injuries sustained (i.e. head injuries, blast, damage to lungs, fractures).

The extent and depth of burns can be influenced by the temperature of the object, liquid or gas that caused the burn and the length of time the casualty was exposed to burning.

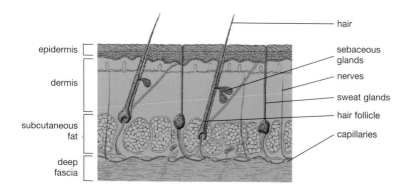

Superficial burns

In a superficial burn, only the top layer (epidermis) of the skin is damaged. A common example is radiation by ultraviolet light producing sunburn. If severe, some fluid may leak into the epidermis causing swelling and blistering.

Superficial partial thickness burns

Superficial partial thickness burns occur when the upper layers of the dermis are injured resulting in leakage of fluid into the tissues, producing blistering. These burns are commonly caused by brief exposure to flame or spill scalds of 50–70°C. The area is red, very painful and blistered with copious tissue fluids.

epidermis

dermis

subcutaneous fat

deep fascia

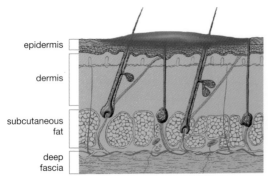 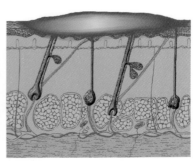

superficial burn (sunburn)   **superficial partial thickness burn**

Deep partial thickness burns

Deep partial thickness burns involve the epidermis and much of the dermis. They are caused by scalds of longer duration or temperature of more than 70°C, or exposure to flame. The area is mottled red and white, dark red or pale yellow, painful, blistered with a moist surface if the blister has broken.

Full thickness burns

Full thickness burns involve the epidermis, the entire dermis and may include deeper structures of fat, muscle and tendons. They may be caused by flame burns, contact with hot metal, immersion scalds, strong chemicals or electricity. The area is white or charred and feels dry and leathery. Because the nerves are destroyed, the pain will not be as great in the full thickness burn with pain at the less burned margins.

epidermis

dermis

ubcutaneous
fat

deep
fascia

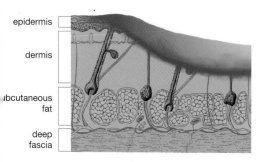 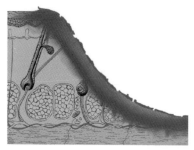

Deep (dermal) partial thickness burn

Full thickness burn

Critical burns

Some burns are classed as critical and include:

- burns that interfere with breathing

- burns where there is serious soft tissue injury or fracture

- burns to the face, feet, genitals, neck, knees, elbows and other areas where the skin folds

- all electrical burns, especially high voltage

- most chemical burns

- burns to young children and the elderly

- burns to people with serious medical conditions such as diabetes, seizure disorders, hypertension, respiratory difficulties.

General principles for managing burns

1 Follow **DRABCD**.

2 Cool the burnt area.

3 Cover the burnt area with a non-adherent/burns dressing (or aluminium foil, plastic wrap, or a wet clean dressing).

4 Prevent infection by covering the burn wound.

5 Minimise shock by reassurance.

Complications from burns

Severe burns

Burn injuries can affect more than just the burnt tissue.
Severe burns also impact on the major body systems.
Complications include:

- shock caused by loss of blood or blood plasma
- infection (the deeper the burn, the higher the risk)
- breathing problems if face and/or throat is burnt or casualty has inhaled smoke, gas or fumes
- circulation restricted or cut off by swelling.

DO NOT   apply lotions, ointments or oily dressings.

DO NOT   prick or break blisters.

DO NOT   give alcohol.

DO NOT   overcool casualty (particularly if young or if burn is extensive).

DO NOT   use towels, cottonwool, blankets or adhesive dressings directly on wound.

DO NOT   remove clothing stuck to burnt area.

When to seek medical aid

Extensive burns

Extensive burns are dangerous and may be fatal—they require urgent referral.

Seek medical aid if:
- the burn involves airway
- the burn involves hands, face, feet or genitals
- burn is deep, even if casualty does not feel any pain
- you are unsure of severity of burn
- a superficial burn is larger than a 20 cent piece.

Types of burns

Thermal burns and scalds

Thermal burns are those caused by heat—contact with an open flame or a hot object; scalding by steam or hot liquid; or burning by friction.

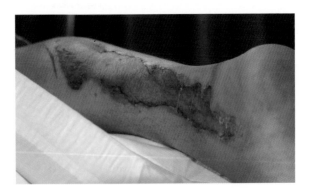

Management of thermal burns

1 Follow **DRABCD**.

2 Extinguish burning clothing—smother with blanket, jacket or use water. If a scald, quickly remove casualty's wet clothing from affected area.

3 Hold burnt area under cold, running water until it returns to normal temperature (up to 20 minutes).

4 Remove jewellery and rings and carefully store and document. Remove clothing from burnt area (unless stuck).

5 Cover burn either with a non-adherent burns dressing, plastic wrap, wet clean dressing or loosely applied aluminium foil.

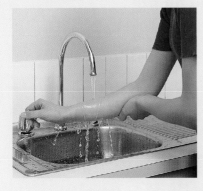

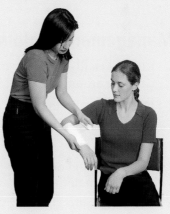

6 Seek medical aid urgently.

Clothes on fire

If a person's clothes catch alight, it is vital to stop oxygen feeding the fire. Stop the person moving or running around as this will fan the flames upward onto face, head and neck. Remember: **STOP—DROP—ROLL—MANAGE**.

If your own clothes catch fire, extinguish the flames by tightly wrapping a woollen blanket, coat or other suitable material around yourself and rolling along the ground. If no suitable material is readily available, don't run around to find material: **STOP—DROP—ROLL**.

Management of clothing on fire

1   STOP casualty from running around.

2   DROP casualty to the ground and wrap in a blanket, coat or rug (wool is best; don't use anything made of nylon or other synthetic materials).

3   ROLL casualty along the ground until flames are smothered.

4   MANAGE as for a thermal burn.

5   Seek medical aid.

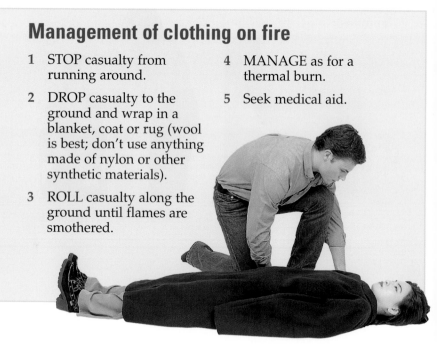

Radiation burns

Radiation burns are caused by radiant energy—energy that radiates from its source. Sunburn is the most common. Radiation burns can also be caused by therapeutic treatment, x-rays, welding equipment, and radioactive material.

Sunburn is caused by overexposure to the sun (even on an overcast day). Some medication can make a person more prone to sunburn. Most sunburn is superficial but in severe cases, the skin may be 'lobster red' and blistered.

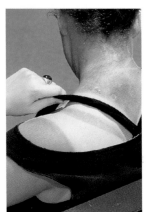

If the eyes are burnt by the sun, they may feel gritty, painful and be sensitive to light.

Management of sunburn

1   Rest the casualty in a cool place.

2   Place under a cold shower, in a cold bath, or sponge with cold water.

3   Apply cool gauze padding to the burnt area.

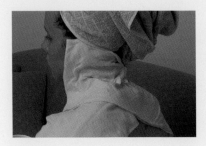

4   Give cool drinks.

5   Seek medical aid for young babies and casualties with blisters.

Sunburn to eyes

1   Cover eyes with thick, cool, moist dressings to cool them and keep light out.

2   Reassure the casualty.

3   Seek medical aid.

Electrical burns

A high voltage electrical burn may be more serious than it appears. It can be quite deep even when the surface skin shows no evidence of burning. High current flow can cause entry and exit wounds where the current density is highest, but most of the damage is to the deep tissues which can be severely damaged by heat. A high or low voltage current flow through the heart, especially alternating current (AC), may cause a cardiac arrest.

Management of electrical burns

1 Check for danger to yourself and bystanders.

2 Switch off power if possible.

3 Remove the casualty from electrical supply without directly touching the casualty, using non-conductive, dry materials (e.g. dry wooden broom handle).

4 Follow **DRABCD**.

5 Wash and cool the burnt area under running water.

6 Apply a non-adherent/burns dressing (or aluminium foil, plastic wrap, or wet clean dressing).

7 **Call 000** for an ambulance.

Note: If the casualty is in contact with high voltage lines, do not approach but wait until power is disconnected by electricity authority personnel.

Chemical burns

Burns are often caused by chemicals used in industry but can also result from chemical agents used in the home. Cleaning solutions (e.g. dishwashing powder, bleach and toilet bowl cleaners), paint strippers and garden chemicals often contain caustic chemicals which can burn tissues.

A caustic chemical will continue to burn while in contact with the skin. Therefore, it is very important to remove the chemical from the skin as quickly as possible.

Chemical burns to the eyes can cause permanent damage and loss of sight. The casualty may suffer extreme pain and be very sensitive to light. If a caustic chemical or acid is splashed into eyes, gently irrigate with running water for 20 minutes (see p. 241).

Management of chemical burns

1   Follow **DRABCD**.

2   If chemical is on skin:

- wash chemical off immediately—use large quantity of water for at least 20 minutes

- remove contaminated clothing and footwear—avoid contaminating yourself

- DO NOT pick off contaminants that stick to the skin.

If chemical is in the eye:

- tilt head back and turn to side

- protect uninjured eye

- gently flush the injured eye with cool water for at least 20 minutes. Keep eye open with fingers if necessary—eyelid spasm may make this difficult.

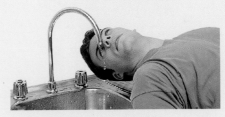

3   Cover the area of eye with sterile or clean non-adherent dressing.

4   **Call 000** for an ambulance.

Bitumen burns

Bitumen burns are normally caused through contact with or
splashing of hot bitumen. It is important that the bitumen not
be removed from the skin unless it is obstructing the airway,
or further damage may result.

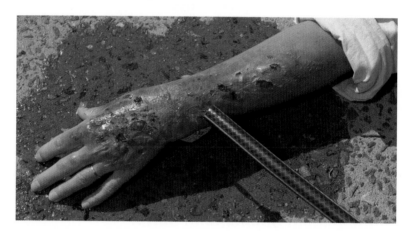

Management of bitumen burns

1   Follow **DRABCD**.

2   DO NOT attempt to
    remove bitumen from
    skin or eyes.

3   Drench burnt area
    immediately with cold,
    running water.

4   Apply cold, wet towels
    frequently.

5   Continue the cooling for
    30 minutes but no longer.

6   If burn is to eye, flush eye
    with water for 20 minutes,
    then cover the eye.

7   **Call 000** for an ambulance.

11

Eye injuries

The eye

The eye is one of the most sensitive and delicate organs in the body. It is easily injured so it is important to treat the eye with great care. Infection can result in later damage to eyesight. Any eye injury can be serious because it can damage the cornea—the transparent tissue forming the circular lens in front of the eye. One rule of first aid for eye injuries is to prevent scratching of or further damage to the cornea.

Eye injuries may be caused by the impact of stones, balls, fists, and other small objects; chemicals (e.g. acids, caustic soda, lime); flames, a welder's flash or ultraviolet light, smoke or lasers; or small foreign objects such as dirt, slivers of wood, metal and sand.

Blows from blunt objects can cause bruising to the eyelids and soft tissue, damage to the bones of the eye sockets, bleeding from blood vessels and even rupture of the eyeball.

Foreign objects can be irritating and cause a great deal of pain and significant damage. The eye tries to flush the foreign object out by producing tears, but this is not always successful. It may be necessary to take further action to remove the object.

Any sharp object which penetrates the eyeball can cause serious damage and may cause infection if not properly managed.

Eye injuries can be prevented by:
- keeping well away from anyone operating machinery at a workbench (e.g. woodturning, metal working)
- wearing eye protection on a building site
- protecting the eyes if there are small objects flying around such as sand or dust
- staying clear of anyone chopping wood or mowing lawns
- wearing protective eye wear when playing sports (e.g. squash)
- wearing a protective shield when welding
- watching out for low branches
- always carrying sharp objects vertically, not horizontally.

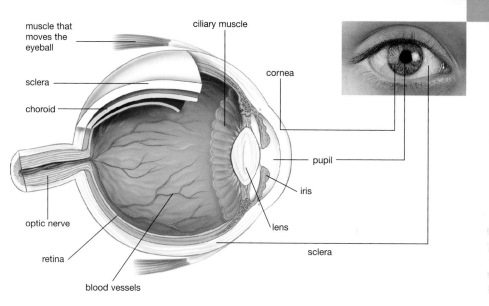

muscle that moves the eyeball

ciliary muscle

sclera

choroid

cornea

optic nerve

pupil

iris

retina

lens

blood vessels

sclera

Eye injuries

So much of what we do and how we operate in our environment assumes the ability to see—loss of sight can, therefore, be a devastating experience. The eye can be injured very easily.

Eye injuries may be caused in many ways—in the home, at work or at sport, in road accidents and by:

- blunt blows
- trauma from fingernails
- cuts from paper
- foreign objects such as dust or grit entering the eye
- damage from burning fluids or chemicals
- the effects of light or radiant energy
- walking into branches.

The first aider has a very important role in ensuring that first aid is given immediately to minimise the chances of partial or complete loss of sight. In a number of cases, it will be necessary to seek medical aid as quickly as possible.

Examination of eye injuries

Inspection of the eye may be difficult because of spasm, swelling, or twitching; mucus and blood discharge; or injuries to eyelid or face.

An eye injury always results in pain and 'watering'. The 'whites of the eye' become red and the casualty may be unable to open the eye.

If the casualty wears contact lenses which can be removed easily, ask the casualty to remove them before you deal with the eye injury. Do not remove the contact lenses yourself. A contact lens should not be removed if the surface of the eye is badly injured.

General principles for managing eye injuries

1 Wash hands thoroughly and put disposable gloves on—remove any powder from gloves by washing.

2 DO NOT attempt to remove an object which is embedded in the eye or is protruding from the eye.

3 Cover injured eye with one or more sterile pads, avoiding any protruding object.

4 Never put direct pressure on eyeball.

5 Seek medical aid quickly.

6 Warn the casualty of a reduced depth of sight perception due to one eye being covered. Vision with one eye only makes it difficult to judge distance. Driving should be avoided.

Burns to the eye

Burns to the eye can be caused by:

- chemicals (e.g. acids, caustic soda, lime, plant juices or sap)
- heat—flames or radiant heat
- welding flash or other ultraviolet light
- glues and solvents.

In addition to the eyes being painful, red and very watery, they will be sensitive to light and eyelids will be swollen. If the injury has been caused by welder's flash, the eyes will feel gritty and painful. This is not felt until several hours after the exposure. The eyelids are often in spasm. Snow blindness is caused by ultraviolet light, and symptoms are the same as those caused by welder's flash.

If chemicals have burnt the eye, act with extreme urgency—within seconds of the injury.

Management of burns to the eye

Chemical or heat burn

1 Follow **DRABCD**.

2 Open eyelids gently.

3 Wash eye gently with cold flowing water for at least 20 minutes (make sure to wash under eyelids–turn upper eyelids back).

4 Place eye pad or light clean dressing over injured eye.

5 **Call 000** for an ambulance as soon as possible.

Welder's flash, snow blindness or other ultraviolet light burn

1 Place eye pads or light clean dressings over the injured eyes.

2 Seek medical aid.

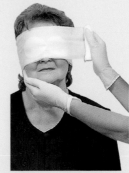

Penetrating eye injury

A penetrating eye injury is usually caused by a sharp object which has gone inside the eye or is protruding from the eye. This injury may cause serious damage and infection if not managed appropriately. If the casualty vomits, the severity of the injury will increase because of pressure caused by the vomiting.

Management of a penetrating eye injury

1   Follow **DRABCD**.

2   Lie the casualty on back.

3   DO NOT attempt to remove object.

4   Place pads around the object or paper cup over the injured eye.

5   Bandage in place.

6   **Call 000** for an ambulance as soon as possible.

DO NOT give any food or drink

lie casualty in comfortable position

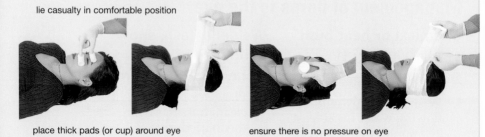

place thick pads (or cup) around eye   ensure there is no pressure on eye

Wounds to the eye

Wounds to the eye caused by a direct blow (e.g. in a fist fight) or by fast moving objects (e.g. a squash ball) can be painful and severe. If the injury is severe, do not persist in examining the eye.

Lacerations and bruises around the eye

Lacerated eyelids generally bleed profusely because of the many blood vessels in this area. A dressing on the injured part will usually control bleeding. However, care must be taken to make sure there is no pressure applied to the eyeball as this may cause permanent damage.

Management of wounds to the eye

1 Follow **DRABCD**.

2 Calm the casualty.

3 Place dressing over injured eye—make sure there is no pressure on the eye.

4 Ask the casualty not to move eyes.

5 Lie the casualty on back.

6 **Call 000** for an ambulance.

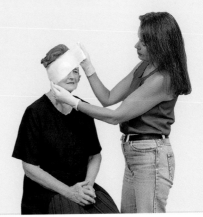

Foreign objects in the eye

Loose eyelashes, grit, dust, glass, cosmetics, metal particles, and insects are some of the foreign objects that may enter the eye.

Warn the casualty of the importance of NOT rubbing the eye, even if the desire to do so is very strong. Rubbing may damage the cornea or other parts of the eye.

DO NOT remove any foreign object from the cornea of the eye, embedded in the eye, protruding from the eye, or persist in examining the eye if the injury is severe.

Management of a foreign object in the eye

If the object is small and is not embedded in the eye, it may be washed out by natural 'watering' (tears).

If tears do not rid the eye of the foreign object:

1 Ask casualty to look up.

2 Gently draw the lower lid down and out.

If object is visible:

3 Remove using corner of a clean, moist cloth, gauze, cotton bud or eye spear.

If object not visible:

4 Ask the casualty to look down.

5 Gently grasp lashes of upper lid.

6 Pull lid down and over lower lid—this may dislodge the foreign object.

If unsuccessful:

7 Wash eye with a gentle stream of sterile saline or clean water.

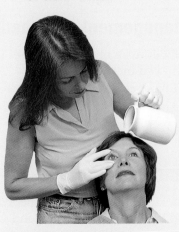

If all unsuccessful:

8 Manage as an embedded object (see p. 246).

DO NOT remove a foreign object from the cornea.

DO NOT remove any object embedded in or protruding from the eye.

DO NOT persist in examining the eye if the injury is severe.

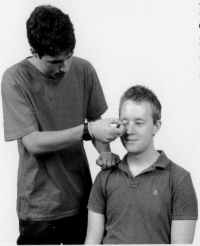

Embedded object in the eye

An embedded object is one that cannot be easily removed by flushing with sterile saline or water. A first aider should never try to remove any object embedded in the eye.

Management of embedded object in the eye

If the foreign object cannot be removed by washing with a gentle stream of sterile saline or clean water:

1 Cover injured eye with an eye pad or clean dressing.

2 Seek medical aid.

Smoke in the eyes

Smoke in the eyes will probably cause the casualty pain and the eyes will look red and watery.

Management of smoke in the eyes

1 Follow **DRABCD**.

2 Ask the casualty not to rub eyes.

3 Wash eyes with sterile saline or cold tap water.

Quick reference to managing eye injuries

Burns to the eye

DRABCD

Open eyelids gently and wash eye with cold flowing water for 20 mins.

Place eye pad or light clean dressing over injured eye.

Call 000 for an ambulance as soon as possible.

Penetrating eye injury

DRABCD

Lie casualty in comfortable position on back.

Place thick pads above and below eye or cover object with paper cup.

Bandage pads in place making sure there is no pressure on eyelids.

Cover injured eye only—DO NOT pad both eyes.

Call 000 for ambulance as soon as possible.

Wounds to the eye

DRABCD

Place light dressing over injured eye.

Lie casualty in comfortable position on back if only the eyeball is involved.

Ask casualty not to move eyes.

Seek medical aid.

Small foreign object in eye

DRABCD

Ask casualty to look up.

Draw lower eyelid down. If object visible, remove with corner of moist cloth.

If not visible, pull upper lid down.

If unsuccessful, wash eye with sterile saline or clean water.

If still unsuccessful, cover eye and seek medical aid.

Embedded foreign object in eye

Cover eye and seek medical aid.

Smoke in the eyes

DRABCD

Ask casualty not to rub eyes.

Wash eyes with sterile saline or cold tap water.

Seek medical aid if necessary.

Head, neck and spinal injuries

The seriousness of injuries to the head, neck and spine cannot be overstated. Once the brain or spinal cord is damaged, the damage may be permanent. The brain and spinal cord do not regenerate after injury—nerve cells are not renewed.

Damage to the brain or spinal cord is one of the most disabling traumatic conditions. Injuries to the head can be complicated by unconsciousness—a sign there is significant brain injury and risk of further injury. Injury to the spine interferes with the transmission of messages to and from the brain, so parts of the body may be paralysed and without sensation.

Any casualty with a head or spinal injury, including injury to the neck, must receive medical aid urgently.

Head and spinal column

Skull

The skull gives the head its shape and protects the brain. It is made up of:

- plate-like bones which fuse together during childhood to form a rigid structure (cranium)
- facial bones which join with the cranium to form the eye and nose cavities
- upper and lower jaws.

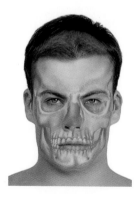
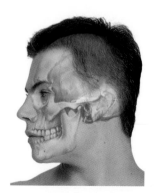

Spine

The spine is a flexible column consisting of 33 small bones called vertebrae aligned one on top of the other. Between the vertebrae are flexible discs which act as shock absorbers for the spine. Each vertebra has an opening in the centre forming a channel from the top to the bottom of the spine called the spinal canal.

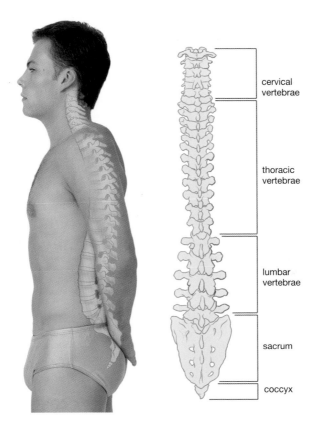

cervical vertebrae

thoracic vertebrae

lumbar vertebrae

sacrum

coccyx

Spinal cord

The spinal cord runs through the spinal canal in the vertebrae and is protected by the spine. It is entirely encased within the spine, floating in watery fluid called 'cerebrospinal fluid' which cushions the stresses of movement. The spinal cord is a continuation of the brain, its nerves radiating out into the rest of the body. The spinal cord and nerves carry messages, as electrical impulses, from the brain to the rest of the body and from the body back to the brain. The spine may be injured anywhere along its length, threatening the very soft delicate structure of the spinal cord.

If the spine is injured, the vertebrae may be fractured and the ligaments sprained or ruptured. Minor injuries may heal without complications. However, severe injuries to the spinal cord itself can result in complete and permanent loss of feeling, and paralysis below the point where the injury occurred. The casualty may become a paraplegic (paralysed from the waist down) or a quadriplegic (paralysed from the neck down). Movement of the casualty with an unstable fracture on the spine may displace the vertebrae further and this may injure the spinal cord.

vertebrae

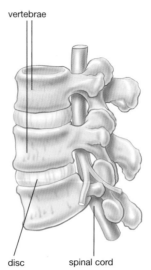

disc   spinal cord

Nervous system

The central nervous system consists of the brain and the spinal cord, both of which are protected by the cerebrospinal fluid. The central nervous system contrasts with the peripheral nervous system which is made up of:

*   12 pairs of cranial nerves arising directly from the brain. These provide vision, hearing, smell, taste, movement and sensation to the head and face
*   31 pairs of spinal nerves running from the spinal cord throughout the body which provide feeling and movement.

The autonomic nervous system, which is part of the peripheral nervous system, controls automatic functions such as heartbeat, digestion and sweating.

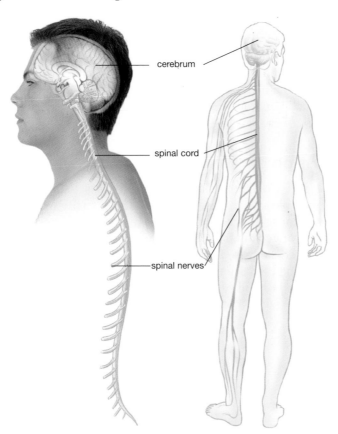

cerebrum

spinal cord

spinal nerves

Head injuries

Because the brain is the controlling organ for the whole body, injuries to the head are potentially dangerous and always require medical attention. When a casualty has a serious head injury, the neck or spine may also be injured.

Warning

If casualty is, or becomes unconscious, suspect a spinal injury. Take extreme care to maintain spine alignment; immobilise as soon as possible.

Fractures

Fractures may occur in the cranium, at the base of the skull, or in the face. The skull may be fractured by a direct force (e.g. a blow to the head) or indirect force (e.g. a fall from a height, landing heavily on the feet). Severe injuries may cause multiple cracking (an 'eggshell' fracture) which may extend to the base of the skull.

Concussion

Concussion is an altered state of consciousness, usually caused by a blow to the head or neck. The casualty may become unconscious but this is often momentary. Common causes are car accidents, falls and sports injuries. The casualty may be dazed, confused and complain of headache and dizziness. The casualty usually recovers quickly but there is always the possibility of serious brain injury.

Compression

Compression is excess pressure on part of the brain. It may be caused by a depressed skull fracture where the broken bones put pressure on or directly damage the brain, or by a build-up of blood inside the skull. If a blow to the head causes bleeding in the brain or on the surface of the brain and the blood cannot drain from the closed space, it builds up and puts pressure on the brain. This is life-threatening.

Assessment of head injuries

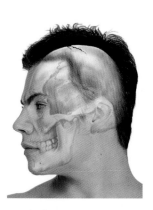

It is often very difficult to make an accurate assessment of the severity of a head injury. Therefore no head injury should be disregarded or treated lightly. As there is the possibility that complications will develop later, the casualty should always be advised to seek medical aid.

The cause of the injury is often the best indication of its severity. Strong forces will usually cause severe injuries to the head and spine (e.g. being thrown through the window of a car in a high-speed accident).

SIGNS AND SYMPTOMS

If the casualty temporarily loses consciousness, but does not have any apparent injury or after effects, the first aider should assume the potential for hidden injury and advise the casualty to seek medical aid promptly. Signs and symptoms of head injury include:

- headache
- loss of memory (amnesia), particularly of the event
- confusion
- altered or abnormal responses to commands and touch
- wounds to the scalp or to face

- nausea, vomiting
- dizziness.

In more complicated injuries, signs include:
- blood or clear fluid escaping from nose or ears. Depending on where the injury is, blood may appear from the ears or nose. If the base of the skull is fractured there may be no obvious sign of injury, but cerebrospinal fluid or blood may escape through the ears
- pupils becoming unequal in size
- blurred vision.

Management of head injuries

1 Follow **DRABCD**.

2 If casualty is conscious, place casualty in a comfortable position with head and shoulders slightly raised.

3 If casualty is unconscious:

- place in recovery position

- clear and open airway

- monitor breathing.

4 Support casualty's head and neck in neutral alignment during movement; avoid twisting movement (could have spinal injury).

5 Keep casualty's airway open with a chin lift, if face badly injured (do not force).

6 Control bleeding but do not apply direct pressure to the skull if you suspect a depressed fracture.

7 If blood or fluid comes from the ear, cover with a sterile dressing (lie casualty on injured side if possible to allow fluid to drain).

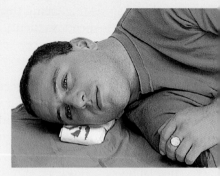

8 **Call 000** for an ambulance. Note the casualty's condition so that you can report it to the paramedics.

Warning

A casualty with a head injury may vomit. Be ready to turn casualty onto the side, supporting head and neck, and clear the airway quickly. You will need at least one helper to do this successfully.

Neck injuries

As the upper spine is part of the neck, all management points for spinal injuries are also relevant for neck injuries. Manage as for spinal injury (see p. 259).

Spinal injuries

A spinal cord injury is particularly traumatic because the resulting damage may be permanent. Adolescents and young adults tend to be the main casualties. Elderly casualties and casualties with bone disease are also at greater risk.

Spinal injuries are always serious and must be treated with great care. Incorrect handling of a casualty can result in paralysis. Careful assessment and management will help minimise permanent disability and increase the casualty's potential for recovery.

Warning

Twisting, compressing or bending an injured spine may worsen damage. Damage to the delicate spinal cord may occur as a result of movement, even if the cord was not injured initially. Take extreme care to maintain alignment of spine.

If the spinal cord is damaged, no messages will be received by the brain or sent to that part of the body below the injury. The control centres for breathing and heart are in the lower parts of the brain. Death may result if these vital cell groups are damaged, or if their messages cannot pass an injured section of the spinal cord.

Remember

After **DRABCD**, swift immobilisation is the highest priority for all spinal injuries.

Causes of spinal injuries include:
- falls from a height
- direct blow to the spine
- penetrating injury such as gunshot or knife wound
- diving or surfing accidents
- high-speed accidents
- sudden acceleration or deceleration injuries (such as whiplash)
- being thrown from a vehicle or motorcycle
- pedestrian being hit by vehicle
- being hit from above by falling objects.

SIGNS AND SYMPTOMS
- pain at or below site of injury
- tenderness over site of injury
- absent or altered sensation below site of the injury (e.g. tingling in hands or feet)
- loss of movement or impaired movement below site of injury.

If the casualty is unconscious as a result of a head injury, the first aider should always suspect a spinal injury.

Management of spinal injuries

Immobilising the spine is the priority for any casualty with a suspected spinal injury.

If the casualty is conscious and medical aid is only minutes away (as in urban areas), place something fairly solid (e.g. an article of clothing, sandbag, padded rock) on either side of the casualty's head to prevent movement of the neck and spine.

If the casualty is unconscious, the airway must be kept open. Remember, airway and breathing always take precedence. The unconscious casualty should be placed in the recovery position, extreme care being taken to maintain alignment of the spine so as to avoid aggravating any possible neck or spinal injury.

Management of an unconscious casualty with a suspected spinal injury (including neck)

1 Follow **DRABCD**.

2 Place unconscious casualty in recovery position supporting neck and spine at all times.

3 Maintain a clear and open airway.

4 Hold head and spine steady with supports, to prevent twisting or bending movement.

5 Apply a cervical or improvised collar (if possible) to minimise neck movement.

6 **Call 000** for an ambulance.

12

Management of a conscious casualty with a suspected spinal injury (including neck)

1 Calm the casualty.

2 Loosen tight clothing.

3 Do not move casualty unless in danger—leave lifting, loading and transporting casualty to qualified personnel (e.g. paramedic) unless absolutely necessary.

4 Support head and neck— place your hands on either side of casualty's head until other support arranged.

5 Hold head and spine steady with supports.

6 Apply a cervical collar if available (a folded towel, newspaper or other bulky dressing can be used if collar not available).

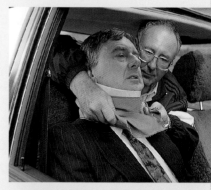

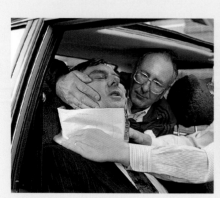

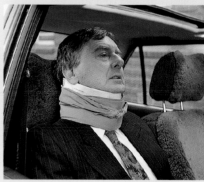

7 **Call 000** for an ambulance.

Remember: Take extreme care at all times to maintain alignment of neck and spine.

Fractures, dislocations, sprains and strains

13

Injuries to bones, joints and muscles are common. Although they are not usually life-threatening, they are painful. If not managed correctly they may cause lifelong disability and deformity.

In addition to the injury to bones, joints, ligaments and muscles, there may also be damage to the major blood vessels and nerves. As a result, there may be blood loss and shock, particularly if there are multiple injuries. Appropriate first aid will reduce pain and shock, and also reduce the risk of long-term complications from the injury.

Ambulance or medical assistance must be sought for all fractures and other injuries when the person cannot move without assistance or is in significant pain. An ambulance should be called urgently, if the limb is pale and cold or lacks sensation following an injury, as this signifies that circulation is reduced.

This chapter includes a description of the functions of bones, joints and muscles and the treatment of different types of bone, joint and muscle injuries.

The musculoskeletal system

The musculoskeletal system is made up of various bones, muscles, tendons, ligaments and joints. It performs a number of functions such as providing support for the body, giving protection to internal organs, storing minerals, producing blood cells (in the marrow) and enabling movement.

Skeleton

The skeleton is the internal framework of the body and is made up of some 206 bones of various shapes and sizes. Its major functions are to provide the anchors for muscles, to support the skin and soft tissues of the body and to protect vital organs such as the heart, stomach and liver *(see human skeleton on p. 491)*.

Bones

Bones are hard, dense, strong structures. They have an ample supply of blood and nerves. Some bones manufacture and store red blood cells in the bone marrow. Calcium is important for bone growth and repair. A lack of calcium in the diet can cause bones to weaken over time, because the body uses calcium from the bones to meet the needs of the body. A decrease in the calcium content of bones from about the age of 60 means bones can become frail, brittle and less dense and, therefore, more susceptible to fractures. This is called osteoporosis.

Joints

Joints are found wherever bones meet. The ends of the bones are held in place by ligaments and by the shape of the bones, themselves. The number and strength of the ligaments determines the amount of movement that can occur. Some joints are highly mobile such as the shoulder, hip and knee while others, like those between the vertebrae in the spine, move only a few degrees. Sometimes the bones are tightly joined or fused— such as the 'joints' between the bones of the skull.

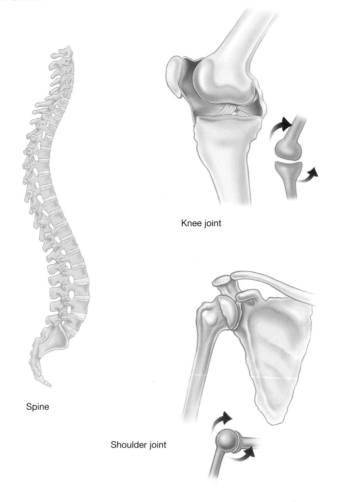

Knee joint

Spine

Shoulder joint

Muscles

Muscles, by contracting and relaxing, work the lever systems of the bones and joints, thus creating movement. Some muscles are voluntary and can be moved at will in response to messages from the brain. Some muscles are involuntary or work automatically to operate the internal organs such as the heart or gut. The skeletal or voluntary muscles arise (or originate) mostly from a bone, usually cross one or more joints and join (insert) into another bone by means of strong fibrous tissues called tendons. By contracting, a muscle moves the bones and changes the position of one or more joints *(see muscle groups on p 492)*.

Musculoskeletal injuries

The bones in our body are built to withstand the many stresses placed on them. They are tough, dense and resilient but they can be broken (fractured) or displaced at a joint. This injury is called a dislocation.

Muscles, ligaments and tendons may be injured by being overstretched. This can result in a sprain of a ligament, a strain (torn muscle or tendon) or a complete rupture. Direct blows can cause internal bleeding in muscles—a haematoma.

Joints are injured when forced beyond their normal movement range.

Note: It can be difficult for first aiders, and it is not their role, to tell whether the injury is a fracture, dislocation, sprain or strain. All these injuries should be treated as if a bone is broken.

Fractures

A fracture is a break in the continuity of bone and is defined according to type and extent. An incomplete fracture —**greenstick fracture**—may extend only part way through the bone, splitting the bone on one side and bending it on the other side. Such fractures occur in children when the bones are soft and pliable. A **complete** fracture is where the bone is broken into at least two parts and may be transverse, spiral, or oblique in appearance. A **comminuted** fracture is one where there are more than two fragments.

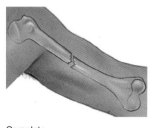
Complete

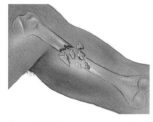
Comminuted

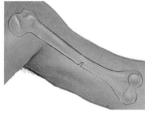
Greenstick

Causes of fractures

Fractures can be caused by either direct or indirect force. The bone can break at the point where it receives a blow—direct fracture, or the force of the blow may travel from the point of impact through part of the body and cause a bone to fracture elsewhere—indirect fracture. For example, if a person falls and uses their hand to break the fall, the force may travel along the arm and cause the collarbone to fracture.

Other indirect fractures can occur when a muscle pulls violently on a bone, separating a fragment. This can occur if a casualty suffers a seizure or when a fast swinging motion is halted abruptly. Rib fractures, for example, can occur because of very severe coughing. Ligaments as well can avulse fragments of bone in sudden twisting injuries, especially around the ankle.

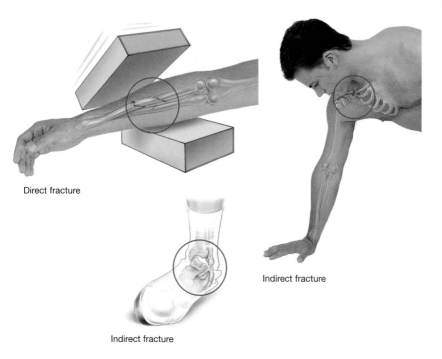

Direct fracture

Indirect fracture

Indirect fracture

Complications

Any fracture can be complicated by injury to adjoining muscles, blood vessels, nerves and organs. Fractures of large bones usually result in considerable blood loss and shock.

SIGNS AND SYMPTOMS

- pain at or near the site of injury
- swelling
- tenderness at or near site of fracture
- redness
- loss of function
- deformity
- casualty feels or hears the break occur
- a coarse grating sound is heard or felt as the bones rub against each other—crepitus.

Fractures are classified as closed, open or complicated.

Closed

When a fracture is closed, the skin over the bone is not broken but there may be bleeding into underlying surrounding tissues. Considerable damage may be done to surrounding muscles and blood vessels and there may be swelling in the affected area because of internal bleeding.

Open

In open fractures sometimes called 'compound fractures', the skin over the bone is broken. In severe cases, the bone may protrude through the skin. There is great danger of infection.

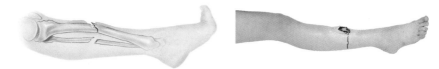

Complicated

Both open and closed fractures may be complicated when there is associated injury to a major nerve, blood vessels or vital organ. One example is when a broken rib punctures a lung.

Remember

No attempt should be made by a first aider to force a fracture back into place.

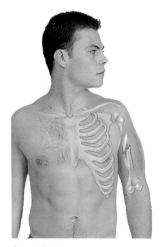
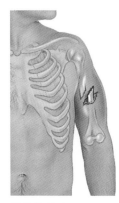
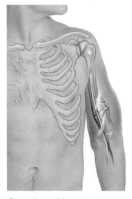

Closed fracture   Open fracture   Complicated fracture

A fracture involving a large bone or causing injury to a vital organ can cause marked distress either from heavy blood loss internally or externally, or from damage to underlying organs.

Aims of fracture management

- Immobilise the injured part in order to lessen pain.
- Reduce serious bleeding and shock.
- Prevent further internal or external damage.
- Prevent a closed fracture from becoming an open fracture.

Splints

Splints are used to restrict or immobilise the movement of an injured limb in order to prevent further injury. General principles are to:

- splint injury as closely as possible to the anatomically correct position
- make sure splint extends beyond the injured area in both directions, ideally to immobilise the joints both above and below the fracture or injury
- apply broad bandages above and below the injured area
- immobilise joints above and below the injured area
- check the casualty's circulation regularly, both in the limb and the rest of the body
- pad the splints to reduce discomfort and prevent further injury.

Management of a fracture

1 Follow **DRABCD**.

2 Control any bleeding and cover any wounds.

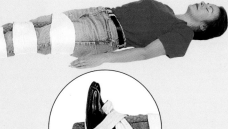

3 Check for other fractures—open, closed or complicated.

4 Ask casualty to remain as still as possible.

5 Immobilise fracture with broad bandages to prevent movement at the joints above and below the fracture by:

6 Watch for signs of loss of circulation to foot or hand.

7 Handle gently.

8 Observe casualty carefully.

9 Seek medical aid.

• supporting the limb—carefully pass bandages under the natural hollows of the body

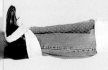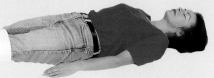

• placing a padded splint along the injured limb

• placing padding between the splint and the natural contours of the body and securing firmly

• checking that bandages are not too tight (or too loose) every 15 minutes.

Note: *If oxygen is available, give up to 8 litres per minute of oxygen if you are trained in its use.*

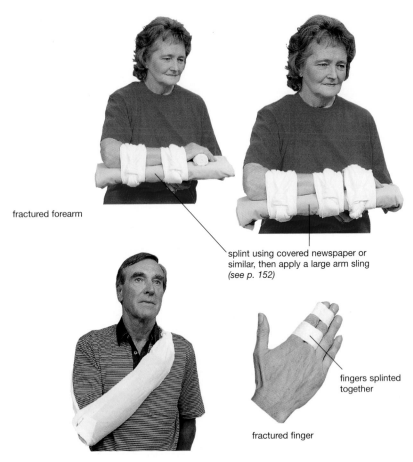

fractured forearm

splint using covered newspaper or
similar, then apply a large arm sling
(see p. 152)

fingers splinted
together

fractured finger

fractured clavicle
(collarbone)
(see p. 150)

Fractures to ribs

Fractured ribs are most commonly seen in elderly casualties
who have falls at home. A simple rib fracture is rarely life-
threatening but is painful. They are seen in sporting injuries
and can be single or multiple. The number of ribs broken
depends on the severity of the blow.

The casualty will usually attempt to ease the pain by supporting the injured area with the hand or arm. Breathing will be difficult and usually shallow, because normal or deep breathing causes more grating of the fractured ends of the rib, and is painful.

Rib fractures may be associated with a wound or severe blow to the chest which can interfere with breathing. Multiple fractures of the ribs cause a loss of chest wall strength (the chest wall is not rigid) so that the rib cage does not move normally during breathing. This is called a flail chest (see p.276), and is life-threatening.

A common cause of this type of injury is a road accident in which the driver is thrown against the steering wheel. The same type of injury can result if the chest is crushed by a heavy object.

Assessing a chest injury

Follow the **DRABCD** Action Plan and obtain a history of the event. Make a careful examination of the chest area if the casualty is having trouble breathing or complains of pain in the chest area, and the possible cause suggests a chest injury. Expose the chest area—try to ensure privacy for a female casualty. Look for signs of broken ribs, local tenderness, a wound, bruises, deformity, blood and abnormal chest movement on breathing. The casualty may look blue or dusky if ventilation of the lung is reduced.

Chest injuries can be open or closed. In an open chest injury the skin has been punctured as a result of either an external object or a broken rib penetrating the chest wall. In a closed chest injury, the skin of the chest has not been broken. Although there may not be any visible sign of injury, there could be serious damage with bruising or rupture to internal organs and tissues.

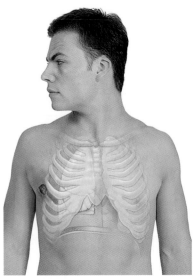

Open chest injury

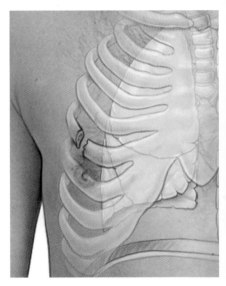

Closed chest injury

SIGNS AND SYMPTOMS

- pain—worsens when the casualty breathes or coughs
- tenderness at site of injury
- short, rapid breathing
- frothy, bloodstained sputum.

Management of fractured ribs

Conscious casualty

1 Place in a comfortable position (normally half-sitting and leaning to the injured side, if other injuries permit).

2 Encourage the casualty to breathe with short breaths.

3 Gently place ample padding over the injured area.

4 Apply one or two broad bandages (depending on size of casualty), securing arm and padding to chest on injured side.

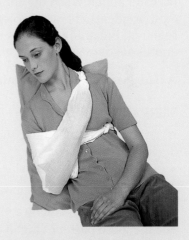

6 If bandages increase discomfort, loosen or remove them.

7 Immobilise the arm using a St John sling or collar and cuff sling.

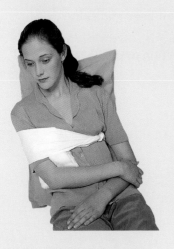

5 Tie bandages in front on uninjured side.

8 **Call 000** for an ambulance.

Unconscious casualty

1 Follow **DRABCD**.

2 Lie casualty on injured side, in recovery position.

3 **Call 000** for an ambulance.

Flail chest

A flail chest occurs when a number of ribs in the same area are broken so that part of the chest is 'floating free'. The injured part of the chest wall is called the flail or loose segment. It does not move with the rest of the rib cage when the casualty breathes. Instead it moves in the opposite direction. This is called paradoxical breathing. If a number of ribs are broken (as can happen when the chest hits the steering wheel in a car accident), the whole breastbone can become a flail segment. Breathing becomes difficult because of the pain and tissue damage.

A flail chest is a life-threatening injury.

SIGNS AND SYMPTOMS

- difficulty in breathing and shortness of breath—gasping for air
- chest pain
- blue colouring of the mouth, nail-beds and skin
- difficulty in speaking
- the loose part moving in a direction opposite to that of normal breathing
- possibly unconscious.

Management of a flail chest

1 Follow **DRABCD**.

2 If casualty is conscious, place in a comfortable position—normally half-sitting, leaning to the injured side.

   If casualty is unconscious, turn to the injured side, in recovery position.

3 Loosen tight clothing.

4 Place a large bulky dressing over the loose area with a firm bandage.

5 **Call 000** for an ambulance.

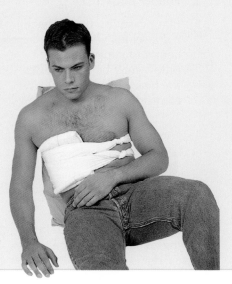

Pelvic injury

A pelvic injury is frequently the result of a car accident, a fall from a height or a crush injury. The casualty will feel pain in the region of the hips or groin which increases with movement. The casualty may be unable to stand and be aware of tenderness or bruising in the groin or scrotum. Signs of shock quickly develop.

Management of pelvic injuries

1. Follow **DRABCD**.

2. Place casualty flat on back if conscious with knees bent and supported—a pillow may be used under the head to increase comfort.

3. Calm the casualty.

4. Remove contents of pockets (they can cause pressure and make movement painful).

5. **Call 000** for an ambulance.

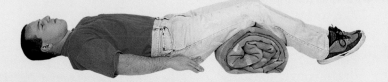

If medical aid will be delayed or you need to move the casualty:

1. Place soft padding between the knees, legs and ankles.

2. Apply a narrow figure of eight bandage around feet and ankles.

3. Apply a broad bandage around knees.

4. Support the pelvis on either side with rolled blankets or sandbags.

Note: : Clothing is not loosened, as this helps to immobilise any suspected fractures in the pelvis area.

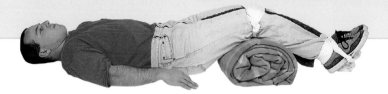

Dislocations

A dislocation occurs when one or more bones are displaced at a joint—most often at the shoulder, elbow, kneecap, and fingers. This occurs when a strong force acts directly or indirectly on the joint and wrenches the bone into an abnormal position. A dislocation can also be caused by a violent muscle contraction.

A dislocation always results in tearing of the ligaments which normally hold the joint in the correct position. At times, the force may be strong enough to cause a fracture and damage nearby nerves and blood vessels.

Some joints, such as the shoulder or fingers, are more prone to dislocation because their ligaments provide less support than those in other joints, which dislocate less easily. A joint which is dislocated may look deformed because the dislocation causes an abnormal lump or depression. A dislocation is always painful and there may also be associated swelling.

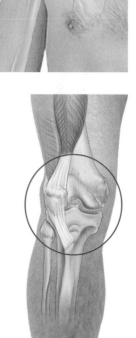

SIGNS AND SYMPTOMS

- pain at or near the site of injury
- difficult or impossible to move the joint
- loss of power
- deformity or abnormal mobility
- tenderness
- swelling
- discolouration and bruising.

Management of a dislocation

1 Follow **DRABCD**.

2 Do not attempt to reduce the dislocation.

3 If injury is to a limb:

- check circulation and if absent move limb gently to try to restore it—**call 000** for an ambulance

- rest and support the limb using soft padding and bandages

- apply icepacks if possible, directly over joint

- if a shoulder, support the arm in position of least discomfort and apply ice compress

- if a wrist, support in a sling and apply ice compress.

Note: If in doubt, manage as a fracture.

Sprains

A sprain occurs when the ligaments holding a joint together are stretched and torn. This happens when a joint is forced to move beyond its normal range. The more severe the injury, the more ligaments will be torn.

Pain from a sprain may be intense and the casualty's ability to move the joint is restricted. There is swelling around the joint and bruising develops quickly.

Management sprains and strains

1 Follow **DRABCD**.

2 Follow **RICE**:

- **R**est the casualty and the injured part

- Apply **I**cepack (cold compress) wrapped in a wet cloth for 15 minutes every 2 hours for 24 hours, then for 15 minutes every 4 hours for 24 hours

- Apply a **C**ompression bandage firmly to extend well beyond the injury

- **E**levate the injured part

3 Seek medical aid.

Note: If in doubt about the injury, treat as a fracture.

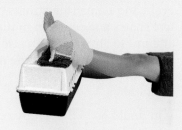

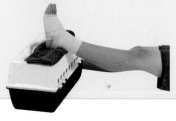

Strains

A strain occurs when the fibres of a muscle or tendon are stretched and torn. This usually happens as a result of lifting something too heavy, working a muscle too hard or making a sudden, uncoordinated movement. Common examples are the groin and hamstring strains of footballers. The casualty will feel sharp, sudden pain in the region of the injury and on any attempt to stretch the muscle. There is usually a loss of power in the affected limb and the muscle is tender.

Remember

If in doubt as to the nature of the injury, always treat as a fracture.

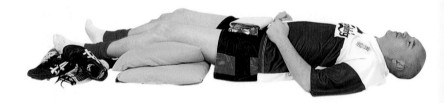

14

Sports injuries

Sports injuries

Australians are renowned for enthusiasm and active participation in a multitude of sports, with participation varying from social or recreational levels through to the more competitive and elite levels. With increasing sports participation at all levels comes increased injury numbers. Most participants are injured at least once during their sporting lives, and many of these injuries could have been prevented.

Each year, around one in 17 sporting participants in Australia are injured sufficiently to miss training or game play, or to seek medical attention. This amounts to approximately one million sports injuries in Australia annually. The football codes, basketball, netball, hockey and cricket account for around 75% of injuries from organised sports and 50% of all sport and recreational injuries. Those who compete on a recreational basis at weekends are more likely to be injured than those competing professionally or semi-professionally, and these injuries are often more commonly seen earlier in the season.

Bruising, resulting from a direct blow, is the commonest form of minor sports injury, followed by strains, sprains and tearing. Knee and ankle injuries are the two most commonly treated sports injuries. Around 20% of knee injuries ultimately require surgery, whilst roughly one quarter of ankle injuries are serious.

As a reflection of increasing sports participation and commencement at an earlier age, an escalating number of injuries are over-use in nature, involving body parts subject to repetitive stress during exercise.

Common sports injuries by sport

Football
- Australian Rules
- Rugby Union
- Rugby League
- Soccer

- corked thigh (painful muscle bruise due to heavy blow)
- muscle strains (e.g. hamstrings)
- head injuries/concussion/lacerations (collisions)
- knee and ankle injuries
- shoulder injuries
- neck/spinal cord injury (becoming less common)

Netball and Basketball

- ankle and knee injuries
- finger injuries and dislocations
- eye injuries (finger or elbow to the eye)

Hockey

- injuries to lower limbs
- injuries from being struck by stick or ball

Cricket

- injuries from being struck by bat or ball
  - bruises
  - head and facial
  - finger injuries/dislocations
- lower back injuries (especially bowlers)

Skateboards/ In-line skating

- grazes and sprains of wrist, knee, elbow
- fractures of wrists, legs, ankles
- head injuries and concussion

Bicycles

- head injuries, concussion, facial injuries
- hand and knee injuries
- shoulder injuries (e.g. fractured collarbone)

Athletics/ Track and Field

- muscle and tendon injuries
- ligament sprains

Jogging

- lower limb injuries
- stress fractures
- heat stress, dehydration

Racquet Sports
- Tennis
- Squash

- knee and ankle injuries
- shoulder and elbow injuries
- eye injuries

Note: Incorrect and/or inappropriate training as well as over-training are believed to account for as many as 40% of all sports injuries.

Sports drinks

Sports drinks are made to a formula that targets the efficient replacement of fluid and fuel during and after exercise. The composition of the typical sports drink is 4–8% carbohydrate (6–8 g per 100 ml), with some sodium and smaller amounts of other electrolytes such as potassium and magnesium. Some newer sports drinks provide a higher sodium level and are designed for athletes in situations in which large sodium losses need to be replaced (ultra-endurance athletes, salty sweaters, rehydration following large sweat losses).

The taste of sports drinks (the combination of sweetness and saltiness) is designed to increase the voluntary intake of fluid during and after exercise, and may help with rehydration goals. However, sports drinks are particularly designed for exercise that will benefit from the provision of extra (carbohydrate) fuel for the muscles and brain/central nervous system.

People who exercise should consider using a sports drink if their event or activity involves at least 60–90 minutes of exercise, and is normally associated with some level of fatigue or deterioration of performance over the course of their activity. An intake of 30–60 g of carbohydrate per hour is a good starting point for experimentation with fuel replacement during exercise, and is equivalent to 500–1000 ml of the typical sports drink.

Fluid requirements during exercise vary according to individual sweat rates, but this range of volumes is also a suitable starting point for most people undertaking sports of moderate to high-intensity exercise. It is not necessary to drink at a rate that replaces all sweat losses during exercise. Rather, people should experiment to develop a protocol for drinking sports drinks that balances fuel intake, the opportunities to drink during their sport, gastrointestinal comfort and the goal of keeping the overall fluid deficit to less than 2% of their body mass (e.g. a 50 kg person should try to drink so that their total weight loss over the exercise session doesn't exceed 1 kg; 2 kg for a 100 kg person etc.).

We are now aware of the need to warn some people against over-hydrating during exercise. Some recreational exercisers manage to drink excessive amounts of fluid during exercise—the combination of low intensity workrate (low sweat losses) and overzealous use of aid stations or fluid intake opportunities is sometimes seen among people at the back of the pack of community marathons or cycling events. Excessive intake of any fluid, which leads to a substantial gain in weight over the course of exercise, can lead to the potentially fatal problem of hyponatremia (low blood sodium levels).

Many people like to drink a sports drink during sports and exercise activities, in which case it doesn't provide a distinct advantage over water—for example, during or after a walk or during a short run or exercise class. This is usually not a problem since it may increase their enjoyment of sport or increase their fluid intake.

Prevention of sports injuries

It has been estimated that 30% of sports injuries can be prevented. This includes 90% of chronic injuries and 25% of acute injuries. The greatest potential for injury prevention lies in:

- education of coaches and trainers
- more adequate preparation and training by players and participants
- warm-ups before, and cool-downs after, sports activities
- increased use of protective equipment (e.g. helmets, shin pads, protective eye wear)
- wearing appropriate footwear (particularly in sports like netball and basketball)
- ensuring sporting facilities, particularly ground surfaces, are of good standard, with padding of goal posts and other hard objects or surfaces

- changing rules that contribute to sports injuries (e.g. changes to scrum and tackling rules in rugby have reduced neck and spinal injuries)
- recognising concussion and not permitting players to resume play until medically cleared to do so
- ensuring all participants are playing at the appropriate standard or age group
- ensuring participants do not resume sport until fully recovered from an injury.

Management of sports injuries

From the first aider's point of view, management of sports injuries is no different from that for the same injury from any other cause.

Having managed the injury, the first aider needs to also consider whether the casualty:

- has other associated (often hidden) injuries
- can continue playing
- should be withdrawn from play.

A casualty should be advised to seek some form of medical advice before returning to play after all injuries except for the most minor of injuries. Following first aid management of a sports injury, it is often up to the casualty (or parents in the case of injury to a child) to ensure appropriate ongoing management. **It is best to avoid:**

H   Heat (e.g. hot shower, heat creams) which increases bleeding and swelling..

A   Alcohol which increases bleeding and swelling.

R   Running (or exercising) too soon which may worsen the injury.

M   Massage in the first 24–48 hours which may increase bleeding and swelling.

If you need to give first aid to someone with a sports injury:

- remember **DRABCD** always comes first
- assess injuries as they occur, not at the end of the event
- consider the possibility of associated (often hidden) injuries
- assess the injury carefully before moving a casualty
- **NEVER** move a casualty with a suspected spinal injury—wait for medical aid
- remember RICE (rest, ice, compression and elevation *(see p. 159)*
- do not offer or allow the casualty food or drink if a serious injury is suspected (e.g. fracture, abdominal injury, concussion).

Abdominal injuries

Abdominal injuries are rare in sport, but are often unrecognised or poorly treated. Such injuries can be caused by blows to the abdomen (e.g. rugby tackle) or by impact from an object at high speed (e.g. surfboard, skiing or cycling injuries).

There is the potential for life-threatening internal bleeding, as the vital organs (spleen, liver, kidneys and intestines) can be ruptured by heavy blows. Casualties may comment on passing dark or blood-stained urine in cases of kidney or bladder trauma.

Management of abdominal injuries

1 Follow **DRABCD**.

2 Check for signs of internal bleeding *(see p. 217)*.

3 If abdominal pain continues, seek medical aid immediately.

4 Do not allow the casualty food or drink if pain continues or if there are signs of internal bleeding.

Air pressure injuries

Air pressure changes that occur during SCUBA diving can result in life-threatening injuries and conditions. Such injuries should be prevented by adequate preparation and training along with strict adherence to safety procedures. This is the basis of requiring a dive licence following completion of an accredited diving course, though injuries may still occur.

Some of the more common air pressure-related injuries include:
- ruptured eardrum
- acute facial pain
- rupture of air sacs in the lung (pneumothorax)
- decompression illness ('the bends'), due to formation of nitrogen bubbles in the blood, which can be life-threatening
- arterial gas embolism (bubbles forming in the blood as a result of a ruptured lung), which can be life-threatening.

Management of injuries caused by air pressure changes

1 Follow **DRABCD**.

2 **Call 000** for an ambulance.

3 Give 100% oxygen if available.

4 Call 1800 088 200 for Diving Emergency Services.

Chest injuries

Injuries to the rib cage commonly occur in the football codes or by direct blows in any sport. The casualty may experience pain over the site of the impact, have difficulty breathing and may be gasping for breath. Rarely, the casualty may cough up blood. In severe injuries, the casualty may collapse. For the management of pneumothorax (ruptured lung) *(see p. 318)* and suspected fractured ribs, *(see p. 275)*.

Stitch

Overexertion or fatigue may result in a cramp (a 'stitch') felt in the lower chest region, deep to the rib margin.

Management of a 'stitch'

1 Ask the casualty to breathe slowly and deeply whilst resting.

2 Seek medical aid if condition does not settle promptly.

Winding

'Winding' or 'being winded' is believed to be a result of spasm of the diaphragm and usually results from a forceful blow to the abdomen or lower chest, or from a fall. The casualty usually gasps and tries to breathe with an open mouth, but the chest does not move air in or out. Whilst this condition settles spontaneously in the majority of cases, underlying abdominal or chest trauma must be considered in cases that are slow to resolve or fail to resolve fully.

Management of winding

1 Rest and reassure casualty.

2 Place casualty in position of comfort to assist breathing (arms above head often helps).

3 DO NOT pump legs or massage abdominal wall (this may cause further damage if casualty is seriously injured).

4 Seek medical aid if no improvement within a few minutes or persisting abdominal or chest wall pain.

Head and facial injuries

Head and facial injuries commonly occur in sports such as cycling, roller-skating and those where there is body contact (e.g. football). Facial injuries may involve the eyes, nose or teeth and may include lacerations and fractures. Depending on the force involved in causing the injury, there may be associated concussion, neck or spinal injury. For management of head injuries see p. 256. For management of other facial injuries see p. 206.

Eye injuries

Eye injuries occur most frequently in the football codes and basketball, but also in racquet sports such as tennis and squash. As a squash ball fits perfectly into the eye socket and is struck at high speed, protective eye wear is essential. All eye injuries are potentially serious and casualties should be referred immediately for medical aid. For management of eye injuries see p. 243.

Fractured nose

Fractures of the nose commonly occur in contact sports such as football, boxing and martial arts, and are usually accompanied by bleeding. The nose may be obviously deformed or deviated to one side.

Management of a fractured nose

1 Assess for associated head injury, concussion and neck injury first.

2 Manage bleeding *(see p. 210)*, sit casualty forward—apply icepacks to back of neck and forehead.

3 Instruct the casualty NOT to blow nose.

4 Seek medical aid.

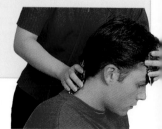

Soft tissue injuries of the neck

These injuries are often associated with swelling and bruising. In severe cases, swelling can result in life-threatening airway obstruction. Spinal injuries must always be considered if a casualty has soft tissue bruising and swelling.

Management of soft tissue injuries of the neck

1 Follow **DRABCD**.

2 If casualty is conscious:

- loosen clothing around the neck—DO NOT remove garments if casualty is complaining of rear neck pain

- apply icepacks to the neck (for no more than 10 minutes).

3 Support neck using a cervical collar or firmly rolled towel or newspaper roll.

4 Observe the casualty carefully for signs of airway obstruction, internal bleeding or voice changes.

5 **Call 000** for an ambulance.

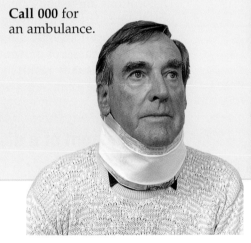

Spinal injuries

Fortunately these injuries occur rarely. Spinal injuries are mostly seen in contact sports such as the football codes, and in diving or surfing. A casualty with a suspected spinal injury should not be moved except in exceptional circumstances (e.g. when there is serious danger or further injury may occur). In such circumstances, great care should be taken and the proper equipment utilised where possible. Where the neck is involved, support to the neck should be applied. A scoop stretcher, *(see p.399)* or similar are appropriate. For management of spinal injuries see p. 259.

Finger injuries

Finger injuries may occur as a result of a direct blow (often 'end-on') or from the finger being stretched out of normal position. These injuries are classically seen in ball-catching sports (e.g. basketball, netball, football and cricket) or contact sports (e.g. boxing and judo).

Fractured finger

For management of a fractured finger see p. 272.

Dislocated finger or thumb

Dislocations are usually caused by overextension, overflexing, or twisting. The joint may be partially or completely dislocated. Partial dislocations may not reveal obvious deformity or gross limitation in range of movement of the joint, whilst complete dislocations usually result in obvious deformity and loss of function of the joint, along with intense pain.

Management of a dislocated finger or thumb

1　'Buddy-strap' the finger to a neighbouring finger as a splint.

2　Apply icepacks to the area and elevate the hand.

3　Seek medical aid.

- DO NOT attempt to put the finger or thumb back in place (bones may be broken).

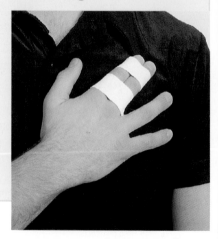

Mallet finger

This is a deformity of a finger due to
rupture of a tendon or a chip fracture
of the base of the end bone of the finger,
near the joint. The finger usually becomes
swollen, painful and the casualty is not
able to properly or fully extend the last
joint of the finger from a flexed position.

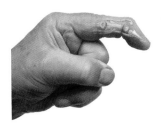

Management of a mallet finger

1 'Buddy-strap' (as for dislocated
   finger above) or splint the finger
   as shown.

2 Elevate the hand and apply
   icepacks to the area.

3 Seek medical aid.

   • DO NOT attempt to straighten
     the finger by traction.

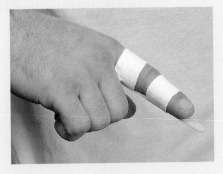

Contusions of fingernails or toenails

Contusions or severe bruising may occur under a fingernail
or toenail when blood collects beneath it, following a blow or
crush injury (e.g. cricket ball to tip of finger). The end of the
finger is often painful and throbbing and bleeding beneath
the nail bed can be excruciating. Underlying bone fractures
or nail bed damage must be considered.

Management of contusions to toenails or fingernails

1 Apply icepacks.

2 Leave nail intact if loose
   or split.

3 Seek medical aid.

14

Ankle sprains

Ankle sprains result in tearing or rupture of ligaments on either side of the joint. First aiders must always consider the possibility of fractures of the bones of the ankle, though this is often difficult to identify.

The injured ankle quickly becomes swollen and bruised, and pain becomes quite intense, in turn restricting movement and resulting in loss of function.

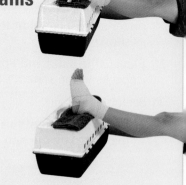

Management of ankle sprains

1   Follow **RICE**:

- **R**est the casualty and the injured part

- Apply **I**cepack (cold compress) wrapped in a wet cloth for 15 minutes every 2 hours for 24 hours, then for 15 minutes every 4 hours for 24 hours

- Apply a **C**ompression bandage firmly to extend well beyond the injury

- **E**levate the injured part.

Note: If a fracture is suspected or you are unsure (e.g. casualty is unable to stand on the injured foot), place padding (e.g. a pillow) around the ankle and seek medical aid.

Blisters

Blisters are caused by excessive friction to the skin and usually occur on the feet, in association with activities such as hiking and jogging. They may also occur on the hands of racquet sport participants or golfers. If friction is felt, it is best to stop activity and tape the exposed area to prevent blister formation.

Management of blisters

1. Put on clean protective gloves to minimise infection risk.

2. Clean the blister area with saline.

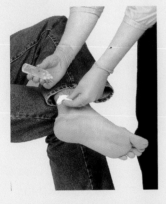

3. Puncture the edge of the blister at 2 or 3 places with a sterile point.

4. Gently express fluid without breaking or removing the skin surface of the blister.

5. Cover with a sterile non-adhesive dressing.

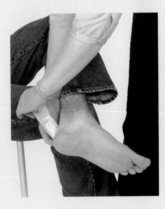

6. Apply surround padding and tape.

7. Seek medical aid if the area becomes reddened, warm or painful.

Knee injuries

Knee injuries are common in sport. Injuries may be from direct blows to the knee region for example, from an opponent falling across the knee or from a fall to the ground. There may be a twisting component to the injury. Immediate first aid has been shown to limit swelling, pain and loss of function, in turn shortening recovery time.

Management of knee injuries

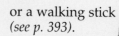
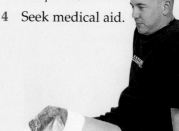

1   Follow RICE *(see p. 296)*; avoid HARM—heat, alcohol, running (exercise) and massage *(see p.288)*.

2   Splint where necessary *(see p. 270)*.

3   Assist the casualty to walk using a human crutch, simple crutches or a walking stick *(see p. 393)*.

4   Seek medical aid.

Muscle cramp and strain

Muscle cramps are spasms or abnormal muscle contractions. There are many possible causes, including overuse, fatigue, small muscle tears, dehydration or poor blood supply to the area. The casualty feels pain, is unable to use the affected muscles and the muscles may stiffen with contraction.

Management of muscle cramps

1   Gently stretch the muscle fully.

2   Apply icepacks.

3   Massage gently if this assists in relieving pain.

4   Encourage hydration/drinking.

Muscle strain

A muscle strain occurs if it is stretched beyond its normal limit. This can result in a stretched or torn muscle. Appropriate first aid has been shown to limit swelling and shorten recovery time.

Management of muscle strains

Follow RICE (see p. 296); avoid HARM—heat, alcohol, running (exercise) and massage *(see p.298)*.

Shoulder injuries

All shoulder injuries should be managed as for a fracture or dislocation *(see p. 280)*.

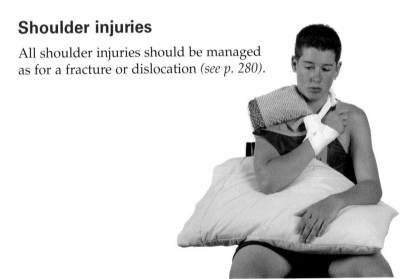

'Corked' thigh (quadriceps contusion or 'charley horse')

A corked thigh is usually caused by a direct blow to the front or outer thigh muscles. It results in bleeding into the muscles and subsequent pain and tightness with muscle contraction. Any stretching causes further bleeding.

Management of a 'corked' thigh

1 Follow RICE *(see p. 296)*; avoid HARM—heat, alcohol, running (exercise) and massage *(see p.288)*.

2 Do not stretch the muscles.

3 Seek medical aid.

Note: Anti-inflammatory medications are not advisable in the first 48 hours as they may increase bleeding. Seek medical advice before considering their use.

Groin and testicle injuries

Injuries to the groin or genitals/testes can occur as a result of direct blows, straddle-type injuries such as in cycling or gymnastics, or by overstretching muscles of the groin or upper thigh. These injuries are often associated with severe pain and in the case of testicular injury, nausea and vomiting can occur. The testes should be protected if playing sports which use hard balls (e.g. cricket), although pain is often still severe despite the protection against more serious injury from blows.

Management of groin and genital injuries

1 Lay casualty on back with knees slightly bent and legs elevated for comfort.

2 Apply a cold compress for groin injuries.

3 Rest and reassure casualty.

4 Seek medical aid.

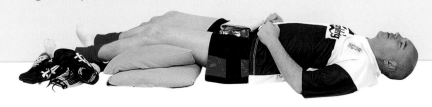

Stress fractures

Repetitive overuse can lead to stress fractures, which are a breakdown of the outer shell (cortex) of the bone. Stress fractures are most commonly seen in runners or participants of sports involving a great deal of running, jumping or prolonged forced walking and are most commonly found in the shin bone (tibia) and the long bones of the foot. Signs and symptoms include tenderness and pain at the site of the stress fracture.

Management of stress fractures

1 Avoid painful activities.

2 Seek medical aid.

Tennis elbow

Tennis elbow is a strain of the muscles and tendons spanning the outside of the elbow joint as a result of overuse. The tendons become overstressed and this condition may (and frequently does) become prolonged. It occurs in many sports (e.g. tennis, squash and baseball) and usually affects the outer side of the elbow. A similar, albeit less common condition called 'Golfer's Elbow' occurs on the inner side of the elbow. Pain and tenderness are usually made worse by contracting or stretching the affected muscles.

Management of tennis elbow

1 Apply icepacks to the outer elbow (excessive ice to inner elbow may damage nerves).

2 Seek medical aid.

Medical emergencies

Medical emergencies

People live with conditions such as asthma, diabetes and epilepsy without a noticeable effect on their lifestyles. However, a medical emergency can arise unexpectedly from complications of these disorders. The cause is not always immediately evident. In such an emergency, the first aider will respond using the **DRABCD** Action Plan and appropriate care.

It is often difficult for the first aider to decide when to send for emergency medical help. If the problem does not resolve itself quickly or you have doubts about its severity, it is better to err on the side of caution and **call 000** for an ambulance.

If you are faced with someone who suddenly suffers chest pain, a diabetic emergency, has an epileptic or other seizure, faints, or has an asthma attack, some general guidelines should be followed.

General principles for management of medical emergencies

1 Follow **DRABCD**.

2 Prevent further injury.

3 Monitor signs of life.

4 When necessary—**call 000** for an ambulance.

5 Provide reassurance.

6 Provide any specific care that will help the condition.

7 Help the casualty to rest comfortably.

Casualties may have items with them which give vital clues about the emergency. Medical warning items such as a Medic-Alert® bracelet, puffer, an EpiPen® can all be clues as to what has caused the emergency.

Medic-Alert® bracelet

A Medic-Alert® bracelet or similar gives information about medical condition.

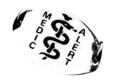

Asthma

A puffer or inhaler is often carried by people with who suffer from asthma.

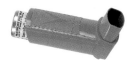

Allergies

EpiPen® —a self injector containing adrenaline indicates a tendency to allergic reactions.

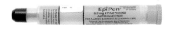

Diabetes

An insulin injector or blood glucose meter carried by diabetics. Sugar lumps or sweets may also indicate diabetes.

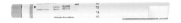

Medication

Glyceryl trinitrate (e.g. Anginine) is taken for angina; phenytoin for epilepsy; indigestion or antacid tablets may indicate a stomach ulcer.

Diabetes

Diabetes is caused by a disorder of the pancreas. In the digestive process, the body breaks foods down into sugars which are absorbed into the bloodstream. In a healthy person, the pancreas then produces insulin to convert this sugar into energy. In diabetes, insulin production and function are impaired. Sugar builds up in the blood, and the cells don't get the energy they need.

The term diabetes covers a range of closely related conditions including:

- **'Type 1 diabetes'** (formerly known as insulin-dependent diabetes)—thought to be caused by an auto-immune process which causes a loss of insulin production. All such patients need insulin to survive.

- **'Type 2 diabetes'** (formerly known as non-insulin dependent diabetes or mature onset diabetes)—is associated with factors such as obesity, common in Western lifestyles; and genetic factors. Dietary control, medication and insulin may be used in management.

People with diabetes may require regular insulin or other medication and must carefully monitor diet and exercise.

Most patients suffering from diabetes use a glucometer—a battery-powered instrument used to collect a drop of blood and to measure the blood glucose level.

Diabetic emergencies

A diabetic emergency may result from too much or too little insulin in the blood. There are two types of diabetic emergency—very low blood sugar (hypoglycaemia, usually due to excessive insulin); or very high blood sugar (hyperglycaemia, due to insufficient insulin).

The more common emergency is hypoglycaemia. This can result from too much insulin or other medication, not having eaten enough of the correct food, unaccustomed exercise or a missed meal. It can develop quickly and some people may not be aware of the early signs.

SIGNS AND SYMPTOMS

If caused by low blood sugar, the person may:
- feel dizzy, weak, trembly and hungry
- look pale and have a rapid pulse
- be sweating profusely
- be numb around lips and fingers
- appear confused or aggressive
- be unconscious.

If caused by high blood sugar, the person may:
- be excessively thirsty
- have a frequent need to urinate
- have hot dry skin, a rapid pulse, drowsiness
- have the smell of acetone (like nail polish remover) on the breath
- appear confused (especially elderly)
- be dizzy or faint
- be unconscious.

Note: *If unsure whether the attack is caused by low or high blood sugar, give a sweet (sugar-containing) drink. Do not use 'diet' soft drinks. Giving any form of sugar can save a person's life. This could save the person's life, if blood sugar is low; and will not cause undue harm if blood sugar is high.*

Although you may not be able to determine the type of diabetic emergency or be able to find out from the casualty, it is important that you recognise the casualty's condition as an 'emergency' and quickly get medical aid.

Management of a diabetic emergency

Caused by low blood sugar

If casualty is unconscious:

1 Follow **DRABCD**.

2 Give nothing by mouth.

3 **Call 000** for an ambulance.

If casualty is conscious:

1 Give sugar, glucose or a sweet drink (e.g. soft drink or cordial—DO NOT use 'diet'soft drinks or diabetic-type cordials—as these do not contain sugar).

2 Continue giving sugar every 15 minutes until medical aid arrives or casualty recovers—follow up with a sandwich or other food.

3 Loosen tight clothing.

4 Seek medical aid if required.

Caused by high blood sugar

If casualty is unconscious:

1 Follow **DRABCD**.

2 Give nothing by mouth.

3 **Call 000** for an ambulance.

If casualty is conscious:

1 Allow casualty to self-administer insulin (DO NOT administer it yourself, but help if needed).

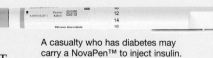

A casualty who has diabetes may carry a NovaPen™ to inject insulin.

2 Seek medical aid if required. If help is delayed, encourage the casualty to drink sugar-free fluids.

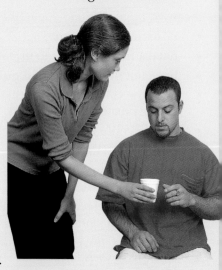

Allergic reactions

An allergic reaction occurs when the immune system reacts to something in the environment that usually doesn't bother people. People can have allergic reactions to medication, insect stings, dust mite, pets, pollens, mould, foods and chemicals. Hay fever is the commonest form of allergic reaction. An allergic reaction can be mild, causing eczema or watery eyes; or may result in severe wheezing or stridor (high pitched sound), requiring immediate emergency treatment.

A severe allergic reaction (anaphylaxis) may be fatal and therefore needs urgent medical attention. Such a serious reaction may cause blood pressure to fall dramatically and breathing to be impaired (anaphylactic shock). The face, tongue and neck may become swollen, increasing the risk of suffocation, and the amount of oxygen reaching the vital organs (heart, lungs and brain) is severely reduced.

Note: For more information call Anaphylaxis Australia on 1300 728 000 or visit: www.allergyfacts.org.au

SIGNS AND SYMPTOMS OF MILD TO MODERATE ALLERGIC REACTION

- tingling of mouth
- swelling of lips, eyes and face
- hives, body rash, itching
- vomiting and/or abdominal pain.

SIGNS OF SEVERE ALLERGIC REACTION (ANAPHYLAXIS)

- difficulty and/or noisy breathing
- wheeze or persistent cough
- difficulty talking or hoarse voice
- swelling/tightness of the throat
- swelling of the tongue
- young children may become pale and floppy
- loss of consciousness or collapse.

Management of severe allergic reaction

1   Follow **DRABCD**.

2   Ask casualty if they are carrying an adrenaline auto injector called an EpiPen®. If so, where State and Territory legislation permits, administer the EpiPen®. *(Ref: www.allergy.org.au)*

Note: *Check with your State or Territory Department of Health for their local laws.*

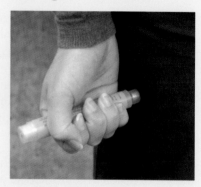

3   Remove the grey cap—this arms the unit ready for use.

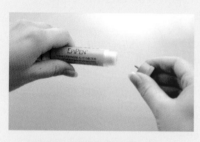

4   Hold EpiPen® in your fist with clenched fingers wrapped around it. Press the black tip gently against skin of the outer mid-thigh.

5   Push hard until a loud 'click' is heard—hold in place for 10 seconds, then remove pen (be careful of the needle that will now be projecting).

6   Massage the injection area for 10 seconds.

7   **Call 000** for an ambulance.

8   Keep the casualty in a sitting or lying position; do not allow casualty to stand as this may result in a sudden drop in blood pressure and a loss of consciousness.

9   Observe and record pulse and breathing.

10 If casualty is conscious:

   • help casualty to sit in a position that most relieves breathing difficulty.

   • Follow **DRABCD**.

Asthma

Asthma is a condition in which the bronchi (air tubes of the lungs) go into spasm and become narrower. Excess mucus is produced, causing the person to have difficulty breathing. Asthma is particularly common in children.

Factors triggering an asthma attack may include:

- exercise
- respiratory infections
- allergies (e.g. to pollens, foods, bee sting)
- exposure to a sudden change in weather conditions, especially cold air
- anxiety or emotional stress
- house dust
- smoke
- certain food additives or preservatives.

Trigger factors may lead to inflammation, narrowing and excess mucus production in the airways. This causes asthma symptoms of wheezing, chest tightness, shortness of breath and cough. Not all symptoms may occur.

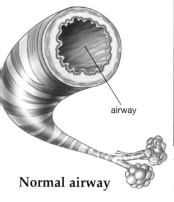

airway

Normal airway

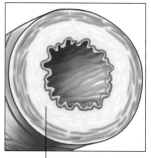

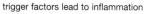

trigger factors lead to inflammation

Asthma affected airways

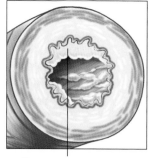

swelling and mucus in airway

SIGNS AND SYMPTOMS

The casualty may be:

- unable to get enough air
- progressively more anxious, short of breath, subdued or panicky
- focused only on breathing
- coughing, wheezing
- pale, sweating
- blue around lips, ear lobes and fingertips
- unconscious.

Note: *A wheeze may be audible. However, in a severe attack there may be so little air movement that a wheeze may not be heard.*

If breathing does not become easier soon after medication—say within 4 minutes, or the attack increases in severity, call for medical aid.

Medication

Asthmatics use two types of medication—relievers and preventers, usually administered by an inhaler.

Relievers

Relievers open the narrowed airways. They act within seconds or minutes. First aiders are primarily involved with relievers in the acute or emergency situation. If an asthma attack occurs, prompt administration of a reliever inhaler containing medication such as Ventolin, Airomir, Asmol, Epaq or Bricanyl is given to provide relief. This medication is usually in a blue or grey container. Relievers reduce the muscle spasm and open the bronchi to allow oxygen to be taken up.

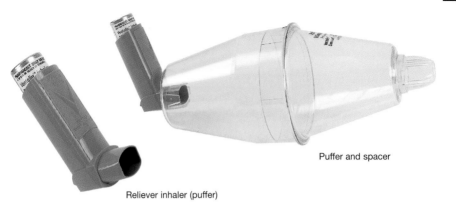

Puffer and spacer

Reliever inhaler (puffer)

Preventers

Preventers such as Pulmicort, Flixotide, Alvesco, Ovar, Singulair, reduce the inflamation in the airways and reduce symptoms and exacerbations. They are usually in a brown or yellow container. This form of medication must be taken regularly to prevent asthma attacks.

Combination medication

Many people with asthma take a combination medication (Seretide, Symbicort) which is a preventer plus a symptom controller (long-acting beta agonist) in the same puffer.

Administration

These medications are given via a puffer or metered dose inhaler—a small pressure canister which releases a regulated dose into the mouth when the canister is pressed. Sometimes a puffer is used in conjunction with a spacer device. Medication may also be given through other devices (e.g. Turbuhaler, Autohaler, Accuhaler or Nebuliser), which also release a regulated dose.

Management of an asthma attack

1 Follow **DRABCD**.

2 Assist the casualty, if conscious, into a comfortable position—usually sitting upright and leaning forward. Do not leave casualty.

3 Be reassuring and ensure adequate fresh air.

4 Assist with prompt administration of medication:

- give 4 puffs of a blue or grey reliever inhaler (puffer)

- casualty takes a breath with each puff, use a spacer if available—give 4 puffs one at a time; casualty takes 4 breaths after each puff—wait 4 minutes

- if no improvement, give another 4 puffs.

5 If little or no improvement within minutes—**call 000** for an ambulance.

6 Keep giving 4 puffs every 4 minutes until ambulance arrives:

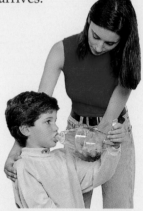

- children 4 puffs each time is a safe dose

- adults up to 6–8 puffs every 5 minutes may be given for a severe attack while waiting for the ambulance.

7 If casualty is unconscious, follow **DRABCD**.

Call 000 for an ambulance immediately.

Where permitted under local State or Territory regulations:

- use another person's reliever inhaler, or use one from a first aid kit to assist a casualty with a severe asthma attack

- if someone is having difficulty breathing, but has not previously had an asthma attack, assist in giving 4 puffs of a reliever and continue with 4 puffs every 4 minutes if required, until an ambulance arrives.

Living with asthma

Although asthma is treatable and usually can be managed well, there is no known cure.

Asthma can affect people differently. Recognising and treating symptoms early can reduce the severity of an attack.

Assessing the severity of an asthma attack

Mild	Moderate	Severe *
• cough, soft wheeze • minor difficulty breathing • no difficulty speaking in sentences	• persistent cough, loud wheeze • obvious difficulty breathing • able to speak in short sentences	• very distressed, anxious • gasping for breath • able to speak only a few gasping words in only one breath • pale and sweaty • may have blue lips

Warning *

Anyone having a SEVERE asthma attack needs URGENT medical treatment. **Call 000** for an ambulance.

Successful asthma management aims at prevention of symptoms, so that the person's lifestyle is unaffected. All people with asthma should develop a written Asthma Action Plan with their own doctor.

Exercise-induced asthma

Most people who suffer from asthma do not have a written Asthma Action Plan. The majority of people who have asthma lead normal lives. Many take part in normal exercise and/or competitive sport. During exercise the airways dry out, due to an increased air intake, increasing susceptibility to an attack. There can be a great deal of variation from day to day in the occurrence and severity
of asthma, although it is known that:

- an attack is more likely after 6–8 minutes of vigorous exercise, especially in a dry cool climate
- symptoms can occur soon after exercise (in cool-down period), and may be at their worst 5–10 minutes after exercise, as well as during activity.

People with asthma should exercise prudently to improve their general fitness and lung function.

However, they should avoid exercise when:
- they have a viral infection
- symptoms of asthma are already apparent
- a known allergen (e.g. pollen) is present.

If asthma is well controlled, exercise-induced asthma is unlikely, so people with asthma should maintain good asthma control by following their written Asthma Action Plan and visit their doctor regularly.

If exercise-induced asthma occurs, the doctor should advise on the appropriate strategies such as:
- use of blue reliever 5–10 minutes before they exercise
- use of symptom controllers (Oxis, Serevent, Foradile) and some preventers such as (Intal Forte, Tilade or Singulair) may also be used before exercise

- a warm-up:
  - 2–3 minute jog, followed by a 30 second sprint, then
    1 minute rest (repeat sprint/rest cycle 5–7 times)

  or
  - a brisk walk or slow jog of 20–30 minutes
  - stretching exercises.

Care of a puffer (metered dose inhaler)

1   Remove medication cylinder from inhaler.

2   Wash plastic inhaler in warm, soapy water.

3   Clear nozzle hole of residue (inside inhaler).

4   Rinse inhaler in clean water and air dry.

Other devices like the Turbuhaler should not be washed—
always read the manufacturer's instructions.

Care of a spacer

1   Remove puffer from spacer.

2   Wash spacer in warm water with kitchen detergent.

3   Drain and air dry—do not rinse.
    DO NOT use a cloth to dry spacer.

*Note: Some spacers are dishwasher safe. Always follow the
manufacturer's advice.*

Spontaneous pneumothorax

A closed or spontaneous pneumothorax may happen in otherwise healthy people without any apparent cause. It can be the result of a violent bout of coughing, a severe asthma attack, or a serious lung infection. The effect is similar to the collapse of a lung due to it being pierced by a broken rib.

SIGNS AND SYMPTOMS

- pain (often under the shoulderblade) on the affected side, worse when the casualty breathes
- difficulty breathing
- restricted or no movement of chest wall on the affected side
- rapid, weak pulse
- duskiness (cyanosis) of the skin.

A pneumothorax can involve the collapse of one or both lungs, resulting in a life-threatening situation. The first aider cannot stop the build-up of air in the pleural cavity.

Management of a spontaneous pneumothorax

1 Follow **DRABCD**.

2 **Call 000** for an ambulance.

3 Make the casualty as comfortable as possible.

4 Calm the casualty.

5 Complete the initial assessment.

6 Monitor vital signs.

7 Give oxygen therapy if qualified to do so.

8 Give emergency care as required.

Hyperventilation

Hyperventilation is a result of involuntary over-breathing.
It can be due to excitement, hysteria, stress or other emotion
(e.g. at a rock concert). Rate and depth of breathing are more than
is necessary to maintain normal levels of carbon dioxide in the
blood. Consequently, carbon dioxide in the blood falls, causing a
range of symptoms. Signs may include shallow, rapid breathing,
rapid pulse, feeling of suffocating, dizziness, pins and needles,
tingling or dramatic involuntary spasms of hands and feet.

Management of emotive hyperventilation

1   Follow **DRABCD**.

2   Calm casualty and remove
    to a quiet, private place.

3   Encourage slow, regular
    breathing—slowly count
    breaths aloud.

4   Seek medical aid.

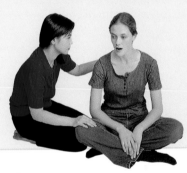

Smoke and gas inhalation

Inhalation of smoke, gas or toxic fumes can cause a respiratory
emergency. A flue leak (e.g. from a stove, heater) can cause the
carbon monoxide level in a room to become dangerously high.
Inhalation of smoke can reduce the amount of oxygen getting
to the lungs and also cause swelling and burning of the airway.
The casualty may inhale dangerous levels of toxic fumes
(e.g. from burning plastic furniture, paint, thinners, petroleum
products and adhesives), especially in confined or insufficiently
ventilated spaces. This can result in loss of consciousness
and death.

An inhalation injury must always be considered a life-
threatening emergency. It is important to ensure that the
casualty receives medical help as quickly as possible.

Warning

It may be some hours before the effect of inhaling toxic fumes interferes with a person's breathing.

Management of inhalation emergency

1   Follow **DRABCD**.

2   Remove casualty from smoke or toxic atmosphere—if safe.

3   Sit casualty upright and loosen tight clothing.

4   **Call 000** for an ambulance.

5   Administer oxygen if available, and you are trained in its use.

6   If breathing stops, commence CPR.

7   If casualty has obvious difficulty in breathing and a wheeze, consider the use of a reliever inhaler (puffer) if available (see p. 312 for use of a reliever inhaler).

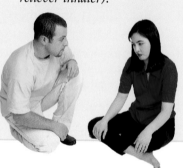

Strangulation

The casualty may be conscious or unconscious.

Management of strangulation and hanging

1   If casualty hanging, support weight of body.

2   Remove any constricting material/free neck from noose.

3   Follow **DRABCD**.

4   **Call 000** for an ambulance.

Cardiovascular emergencies

Cardiovascular disease is one of the four 'big killers' in Australia—the others being stroke, cancer and injury.

Chest pain or discomfort is an important symptom. However, not all chest pain and discomfort is caused by cardiovascular disease. Some chest pain results from less serious conditions. Conversely, not all heart emergencies are accompanied by serious chest pain or discomfort.

Cardiovascular disorders

Cardiovascular disease (diseases of the heart and circulatory system) can develop from an early age. Life-long inappropriate diet, smoking and genetic predisposition are contributing factors.

Although the proportion of people who die each year from cardiovascular disease has been declining since the 1960s, it is still the number one cause of death in Australia.

Who will develop cardiovascular disease?

Some people are more at risk than others. Men are more likely to develop heart disease than women—although the difference in gender risk decreases with increasing age. Also at higher risk are people of lower socio-economic status, those who have a family history of heart disease, and indigenous Australians. Other factors which increase the risk of cardiovascular disease include:

- obesity
- unhealthy eating
- smoking
- high blood pressure (hypertension)
- disorders of fat in the blood
- diabetes.

When people suffer from a combination of risk factors—such as obesity, smoking and high blood pressure—the possibility of a heart attack or stroke is substantially increased.

Atherosclerosis (narrowing of the arteries)

Narrowing of the arteries occurs when fatty deposits (called cholesterol plaques) build up on the inner walls of arteries. This may remain undetected for years. In the coronary arteries the gradual narrowing of the vessels is called coronary artery disease.

As an artery gets narrower, less and less blood can get through. Atherosclerosis may begin in later childhood although symptoms may not be obvious until middle age or later. Some studies have shown that coronary artery disease which begins in teenage years is associated with a diet high in saturated fats; and is worse in smokers.

Signs and symptoms of atherosclerosis begin when a narrowed section of artery prevents the heart tissues beyond from receiving enough oxygenated blood.

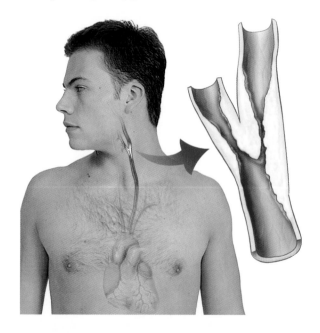

Angina

Angina is temporary chest discomfort or pain that typically comes on with exercise or emotional stress. It usually lasts only a matter of minutes. It occurs because the narrowed coronary arteries are unable to supply the additional oxygen-carrying blood needed when the heart's activity increases.

Angina, also called 'angina pectoris', is usually relieved by rest, and by prescribed medication.

SIGNS AND SYMPTOMS

The pain or discomfort associated with angina is usually described as tight, gripping or squeezing, and can vary from mild to severe. Angina is usually felt in the centre of the chest, but may spread to either or both shoulders, the back, neck or jaws or down the arm and can even be felt in the hands. Sometimes it is experienced in these other parts of the body without being felt in the chest. Sometimes angina is experienced as shortness of breath, rather than pain.

Management of angina

1 Encourage the casualty to immediately stop what they are doing and rest.

2 Help casualty to sit or lie down (whichever is most comfortable) and provide reassurance. Ask them to describe their symptoms.

3 If rest alone does not bring rapid or effective relief of symptoms, assist the casualty either to place his or her prescribed dose of angina tablets under the tongue or inside the cheek as per directions on bottle, or administer Nitrolingual® Pumpspray under the tongue.

4 If symptoms are not relieved within 5 minutes, assist the casualty to take another dose of angina medication.

5 If the pain or discomfort is not completely relieved within 10 minutes of onset by rest and medication, if the pain gets worse quickly, or is severe **call 000** for an ambulance immediately. Don't hang up. Wait for advice from the 000 operator.

6 Stay with the casualty until the ambulance arrives. Monitor vital signs. Be prepared to give CPR.

Note: Give the conscious casualty 300mg (one tablet) of aspirin in water, unless casualty is allergic to aspirin, is already taking anti-coagulant medication (e.g. warfarin) or their doctor has warned them against taking aspirin.

7 If pain settles quickly and the casualty is familiar with their angina, recommend medical follow up as soon as possible.

Heart attack

A heart attack occurs when there is a sudden complete blockage of an artery that supplies an area of the heart. A heart attack usually begins when an area of fatty plaque (thickened with cholesterol) cracks and a blood clot forms over the crack. This blocks the blood flow to the heart muscle beyond the clot and causes the muscle to become damaged.

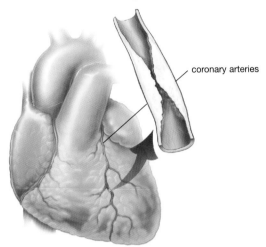

coronary arteries

Heart attack is a life-threatening emergency. The first aider must act quickly and **call 000** for an ambulance immediately because—

1 Damaged heart muscle may initiate an uncontrolled disorganised rhythm (ventricular fibrillation) that may stop the heart beating effectively. This is the most common cause of cardiac arrest. When it occurs, cardiac arrest may follow within minutes of the first symptoms of a heart attack.

2 Paramedics and doctors working in emergency departments use clot dissolving drugs and other treatments which are used to reduce the amount of permanent damage to the heart muscle. These must be given soon after a heart attack occurs to be effective.

If the casualty has chest pain or discomfort similar to angina, but it is not relieved by medication and rest, the first aider should manage the casualty as if he or she is having a heart attack.

SIGNS AND SYMPTOMS

People who have a heart attack usually have some warning signs. The warning signs of heart attack vary and usually last for at least 10 minutes.

A heart attack usually causes discomfort or pain in the centre of the chest. The pain may come on suddenly, or sometimes may start slowly, developing over minutes. The sensation may feel like tightness, pressure, heaviness, fullness, or squeezing. The pain may be severe, moderate or mild. The chest discomfort or pain may spread to the neck and jaw, throat, shoulders, the back, either or both arms and into the wrist and hands.

Some people do not get any chest discomfort – only discomfort in these parts of the upper body. There may be a choking feeling in the throat. The arms may feel 'heavy' and 'useless.' Often there will also be sweating, shortness of breath, dizziness or feeling light-headed and a sick feeling or actual vomiting.

Many people experiencing a heart attack delay seeking care. They do not realise they are having a heart attack or simply associate the symptoms with indigestion or muscle soreness. The symptoms of heart attack may seem, to the casualty, to be simply a sensation of gastric discomfort, like indigestion. To delay treatment is to risk death and disability from permanent damage to the heart muscle, or from sudden death through cardiac arrest.

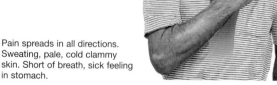

Pain spreads in all directions.
Sweating, pale, cold clammy
skin. Short of breath, sick feeling
in stomach.

Management of heart attack

1 Follow **DRABCD**.

2 Encourage the casualty to immediately stop what they are doing and rest. Help the casualty to sit or lie down, whichever is most comfortable and provide reassurance. Ask them to describe their symptoms.

3 If any of the symptoms are severe, get worse quickly, or last for 10 minutes **call 000** for an ambulance immediately. **Do not** hang up. Wait for advice from the 000 operator.

4 Loosen tight clothing.

5 Give the conscious casualty 300 mg (one tablet) of aspirin in water, unless the casualty is allergic to aspirin, is already taking anti-coagulant medication (e.g. warfarin) or their doctor has warned them against taking aspirin.

6 Stay with the casualty until the ambulance arrives. Monitor vital signs. Be prepared to give CPR.

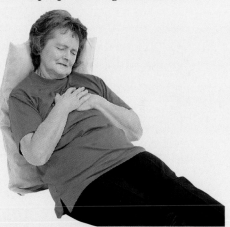

If casualty is unconscious, or if lapsing into unconsciousness:

1 Place casualty on side in recovery position.

2 Follow **DRABCD**.

3 **Call 000** for an ambulance immediately.

Chronic heart failure

Chronic heart failure (also known as congestive heart failure) is an ongoing condition in which the heart cannot pump normally. It usually develops as a result of old age or chronic heart disease.

SIGNS AND SYMPTOMS

- a general feeling of tiredness
- breathlessness when exercising or lying flat
- swollen feet, ankles, legs and abdomen
- coughing and wheezing.

With advanced congestive heart failure, the casualty may feel breathless even when resting and may have to sit up to be comfortable.

Management of chronic heart failure

If casualty is conscious:

1   Help casualty to a sitting position.

2   Reassure and loosen tight clothing.

If the casualty becomes breathless or collapses:

1   Follow **DRABCD**.

2   **Call 000** for an ambulance immediately.

Stroke 'cerebrovascular accident'

A stroke occurs when an artery taking blood to the brain becomes blocked or bursts. In most cases, this is the result of a clot at a part of an artery narrowed by long-term build-up of fatty deposits. As a result of a stroke, brain cells are damaged and functions controlled by that part of the brain become paralysed.

Paralysis of parts of the body or speech problems are common after a stroke. Although many people make a good recovery, a stroke can be fatal.

Sometimes the person will get warnings of a future stroke. These 'mini strokes' (also called TIAs) are due to spasm of the blood vessels, or are the result of temporary blockage in smaller arteries supplying oxygen-carrying blood to the brain. These are associated with the same symptoms as a stroke but are temporary and do not cause long-term harm to the brain. They are caused by temporary disruptions to the brain's blood supply. Seek medical attention as a future stroke may be preventable. People most at risk of a stroke are those who are elderly, have high blood pressure, smoke, have heart disease or diabetes, or have previously had a stroke. A stroke is a life-threatening emergency.

SIGNS AND SYMPTOMS

- sudden decrease in level of consciousness
- weakness or paralysis, especially on one side of body
- feeling of numbness in face, arm or leg
- difficulty speaking or understanding
- unexplained dizziness
- disturbed vision
- loss of balance
- confusion.

Inability to communicate when otherwise alert can cause extreme anxiety in the casualty. Grasp both hands and ask the casualty to squeeze. Usually casualty will respond with one or other hand. Then communicate by hand squeezes—one for yes and two for no. Be calm and reassuring.

Management of stroke

1 Follow **DRABCD**.

2 **Call 000** for an ambulance.

3 Reassure the casualty.

4 If casualty is conscious:

- support head and shoulders on pillows
- loosen tight clothing
- maintain body temperature
- wipe away secretions from mouth
- ensure airway is clear and open.

5 If casualty is unconscious:

- place in recovery position.

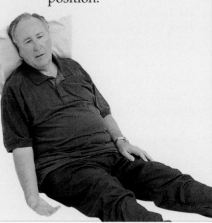

Fainting

Fainting is a partial or complete loss of consciousness caused by a temporary reduction of blood flow to the brain. It can be triggered by emotional shock, pain, over-exertion, exhaustion, lack of food, sight of blood, or in most cases, standing immobile in hot conditions. Some people such as pregnant women, or the elderly can faint as a result of changing position (e.g. from sitting to standing). But fainting can occur at any time. It results in a brief loss of consciousness, slow pulse and pallor.

SIGNS AND SYMPTOMS

The casualty may:

- lose consciousness or feel light-headed
- dizzy or nauseated
- have a pale, cool, moist skin
- have numbness in the fingers and toes.

Usually people recover quickly, often within seconds, without any lasting effects. However, if fainting is the result of an underlying medical condition, the casualty should see a doctor.

Management of fainting

1 Follow **DRABCD**.

2 Loosen any tight clothing.

3 Ensure plenty of fresh air—open window if possible.

4 When casualty is conscious, lie on back and raise and support legs. For a woman in advanced pregnancy, place padding under right buttock to tilt.

4 Treat any injury resulting from a fall.

Note: *Do not sit the casualty on a chair with head between knees.*

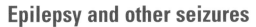

Epilepsy and other seizures

Epilepsy is a disorder of the brain characterised by a tendency to have recurrent seizures and is defined by two or more unprovoked seizures. Seizures may vary from the briefest lapses of attention or muscle jerks to severe and prolonged convulsions. They may also vary in frequency, from less than one a year to several per day.

Seizures are the result of sudden, usually brief, excessive electrical discharges in a group of brain cells (neurones). Sometimes they involve the whole brain, sometimes only part of the brain. The clinical signs of seizures will therefore vary and depend on where in the brain the seizure first starts and how far it spreads. Transient symptoms can occur, such as loss of awareness or consciousness and disturbances of movement, sensation (including vision, hearing and taste), mood or mental function.

Not all seizures are epilepsy. Some seizures are provoked by events such as head injury, high fever, brain tumour, poisoning, drug overdose, stroke, serious infection, or severe impairment of oxygen or blood to the brain. These are not considered epilepsy nor do they result in long-term seizure disorders.

Approximately one in every two hundred Australians has epilepsy. Approximately one in every twenty children will experience a febrile (infantile) convulsion caused by high fever. For management of an infantile convulsion *see p. 334.*

All seizures require first aid care, and the first aider must stay with the casualty. However, if a tonic-clonic seizure (grand mal) occurs, first aid will be needed. A tonic-clonic seizure starts very suddenly but seldom lasts longer than 2–3 minutes. If this is a casualty's first ever seizure, they must go to medical aid.

SIGNS AND SYMPTOMS

A person having a tonic-clonic seizure may:
- suddenly cry out
- fall to the ground—sometimes resulting in injury
- stiffen and lie rigid for a few seconds
- have rhythmic jerking muscular movements
- look very pale and have blue tinged lips
- have excessive saliva coming out of the mouth
- sometimes bite the tongue or cheek, resulting in blood in the saliva
- lose control of bladder and/or bowel
- be extremely tired, confused or agitated afterwards.

Management of a tonic-clonic seizure

During the seizure

1 DO NOT try to restrain the person.

2 DO NOT put anything in the mouth.

3 DO NOT move the person unless in danger.

4 Protect the casualty from injury.

5 Place something soft under head and shoulders.

After the seizure

1 Follow **DRABCD**.

2 Keep airway clear by placing casualty on side in recovery position as soon as jerking stops, or immediately if they have vomited or have food or fluid in their mouth.

3 Manage any injuries resulting from the seizure.

4 DO NOT disturb if casualty falls asleep but continue to check signs of life.

Call an ambulance if:

- the seizure continues for more than 5 minutes
- another seizure quickly follows
- the person has been injured
- the person has a history of diabetes.

Infantile convulsions

Convulsions in infants and children may be due to fever, infection, epilepsy or other conditions. A rapid rise in body temperature, to even as little as 38.5°C (normal is 37°C), can cause convulsions in infants and young children, most often those aged 6 months to 5 years. Often the seizure is the first sign of a fever so it is very difficult to prevent these convulsions. Infantile (febrile) convulsions are usually brief, lasting no more than 5 minutes, and are quite common—one in 20 children experience them.

Note: *Convulsions caused by high temperature are rare but can also occur in adults.*

SIGNS AND SYMPTOMS

- fever
- stiffening
- twitching or jerking of face or limbs
- eyes rolling upwards
- blue face and lips
- stiffness of body with arched back
- unconsciousness.

Management of infantile convulsions

During the convulsion

1   Place the child on their side for safety.

2   DO NOT restrain the child.

After the convulsion

1   Follow **DRABCD**.

2   Seek medical aid.

Note: DO NOT cool the child by sponging or bathing but remove excess clothing or wrapping.

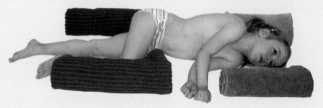

16

Bites and stings

Venomous bites and stings

Animal bites and insect stings are painful and some are potentially lethal. More Australians die each year from bee stings than from shark attacks. Some jellyfish, particularly those found in Australia's far north, are capable of delivering a fatal sting.

Bites and stings occur frequently in the garden, at the beach, in playgrounds and in the home. Most bites and stings are relatively minor but can be often painful. However, others can be deadly, such as bites from a snake (e.g. brown snake, tiger snake or taipan), funnel-web spider and blue-ringed octopus, or stings from the cone shell and box jellyfish. Some stings, especially those from bees, wasps or ticks, can produce a potentially fatal reaction—anaphylaxis.

Venom injected directly into the bloodstream may work rapidly because it circulates quickly around the body. If injected just beneath the skin, the venom will act more slowly because it has to spread locally in the tissue fluids, then moves into the lymphatic system before entering the bloodstream. The venom of most Australian creatures moves in the body's tiny lymphatic vessels. The general effects are slow in onset, as long as the casualty remains still.

DRABCD is the mainstay of management of all envenomation. If the casualty has an allergic reaction to an otherwise non-lethal bite or sting, breathing could be affected and death may result if medical aid is not sought immediately. Be prepared to give CPR.

General principles of first aid for venomous bites and stings

1 Follow **DRABCD**—avoid being bitten yourself.

2 Ask history of event, site of sting or bite and where and when casualty was bitten or stung.

3 Carry out first aid quickly.

4 Seek medical aid—even if in doubt whether the casualty has been bitten or stung.

5 Monitor breathing—be prepared to give CPR.

Management techniques for specific bites and stings

There are four main first aid management techniques for dealing with specific types of bites and stings:

- pressure immobilisation
- cold compress (icepack)
- vinegar
- hot water.

Pressure immobilisation is used to slow the movement of venom from the site of the bite or sting. A crepe or conforming roller bandage about 10–15 cm wide is applied. Improvise with other material if a roller bandage is not available. The pressure immobilisation bandage must be immediately applied over wide areas of the limb *(see p. 160)*. The bandage compresses the tiny lymphatic vessels which carry the venom. A pressure immobilisation bandage, together with splinting, is effective in the management of bites and stings from a:

- snake
- funnel-web spider
- mouse spider
- blue-ringed octopus
- cone shell
- allergic reaction to any bite or sting.

A cold compress (icepack) relieves pain and swelling by reducing the flow of blood to the injured area. The cold compress is usually left on the affected area for 15 minutes at a time and changed whenever necessary to maintain the same level of coldness. Icepacks are available for purchase from St John, or you may wish to make your own *(see p. 159)*. Icepacks or cold compresses are effective in the management of bites and stings from:

- bee
- European wasp
- ant
- non-tropical minor jellyfish.

Another form of management is the immediate use of vinegar for certain jellyfish stings found in tropical areas where the box jellyfish and Irukandji live. Vinegar inactivates the discharge of nematocysts of all known lethal members of the box jellyfish, Irukandji groups, jimble and sea anemone and so prevents further injection of venom.

Vinegar cannot relieve pain from venom already injected. However, application of dry cold (cold packs or wrapped ice) may assist with pain relief.

DO NOT use fresh water on a box jellyfish sting

DO NOT use vinegar on a bluebottle sting.

DO NOT use fresh water on the dried sting from any type of jellyfish as it will cause the undischarged nematocysts to fire.

Hot water is an effective means of treating the symptoms following the injection of venom of some types of venomous marine creatures. The water should be tested to ensure it is as hot (but not hotter) as a rescuer can tolerate before placing the casualty's affected area (usually a foot or hand) in the hot water. This method of management is used for stings from:

- stonefish
- bullrout
- stingray
- catfish
- crown-of-thorns starfish
- bluebottle (Pacific Man-O-War).

Snakebite

Although most people fear snakes, snakebite is not a common occurrence in Australia and the symptoms of a bite are not always dangerous. There are about 100 species of snakes in Australia of which twenty are highly dangerous to humans. The most venomous Australian snakes are the most venomous in the world. Of the remainder, many species are capable of causing moderate to severe symptoms. All snakebites must therefore be treated as life-threatening. Care has to be taken in the bush, in rural areas, and also in suburban areas close to grassland, bushland and rivers. Many casualties who were bitten by a snake are those who were handling the snake.

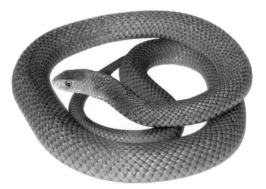

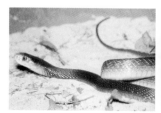

Taipan

Common brown snake

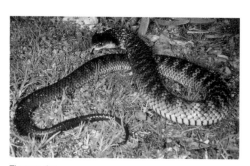

Tiger snake

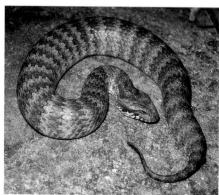

Death adder

Although many snakes (e.g. the pythons) are not venomous, brown snakes have caused the greatest number of deaths in Australia. Several others, including the tiger snake, taipan and death adder, are very dangerous and their bite is always potentially fatal.

Research has shown that the spread of snake venom depends on its absorption through the lymphatic system. If the casualty remains at rest and a very firm pressure immobilisation bandage and splint are applied rapidly (within one or two minutes), very little venom reaches the circulation, even after several hours. Venom affects different parts of the body, but paralysis of the breathing muscles is one of the most serious effects and may lead to death without medical intervention. If a child tells you that they have been bitten by a snake or spider, treat the incident seriously.

Snakes are not normally aggressive and tend to bite only when threatened or handled. However, little or no venom is injected in some bites, and symptoms may therefore not develop. The first aider is not able to assess either the type of snake or how much venom has been injected. As it is not always possible to identify the type of snake, all snakebites should be treated as potentially lethal and medical aid should be sought urgently. All major hospitals have a Venom Identification Kit to assist identification of the snake, which in turn helps in the selection of the correct antivenom.

SIGNS AND SYMPTOMS

Signs are not always visible and symptoms may not appear for an hour or more after the person has been bitten. These may include:

- puncture marks or scratches—usually on a limb
- nausea, vomiting and diarrhoea
- headache
- double or blurred vision
- drooping eyelids
- voice changes

- bleeding from bite site
- breathing difficulties
- drowsiness, giddiness or faintness
- problems speaking or swallowing
- pain or tightness in the throat, chest or abdomen
- respiratory weakness or arrest
- dark urine—due to blood or muscle breakdown products.

Symptoms which can develop up to 3 hours after the bite include:

- limb paralysis
- hypoxia
- cyanosis
- decrease in level of consciousness.

Management of snakebite

1 Follow **DRABCD**.

2 Rest and reassure the casualty.

3 Apply a very firm pressure immobilisation bandage quickly *(see p. 160)*.

4 Splint the bandaged limb.

5 Ensure casualty does not move.

6 **Call 000** for an ambulance.

7 Write down the time of the bite and when the bandage was applied—stay with the casualty.

Warning

DO NOT wash venom off the skin as retained venom will assist identification.

DO NOT cut bitten area.

DO NOT try to suck venom out of wound.

DO NOT use an arterial tourniquet.

DO NOT try to catch the snake.

Spider bites

Some spiders are venomous enough to cause moderate to severe symptoms in humans. Funnel-web spider venom has the potential to kill an adult. Red-back spiders inject venom which acts slowly. Although serious, red-back spiders do not cause death.

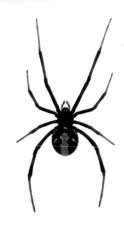

Red-back spider (20–40mm)

Although the Sydney funnel-web spider appears within about 140 km of Sydney, other funnel-web spiders, some of which are potentially dangerous, live in south-east Queensland, parts of New South Wales, Victoria, South Australia and Tasmania. Funnel-web spiders are black or dark brown and 2–3 cm in length. They rear back to bite and have large, strong fangs which can penetrate clothing and bite deeply if the skin is bare. A funnel-web may hang on and in some cases may have to be removed forcibly. The first aider must take care not to get bitten while doing so. This spider's bite can kill a child in minutes and an adult in a few hours if appropriate first aid and subsequent antivenom are not given. However, in many cases there will be very few symptoms.

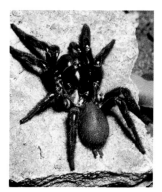

Funnel-web spider (25–30mm)

SIGNS AND SYMPTOMS OF A SPIDER BITE

- sharp pain at bite site
- profuse sweating
- nausea, vomiting and abdominal pain.

ADDITIONAL SYMPTOMS OF A FUNNEL-WEB SPIDER BITE

- copious secretion of saliva
- confusion leading to unconsciousness
- muscular twitching and breathing difficulty
- small hairs stand on end
- numbness around mouth
- copious tears
- disorientation
- fast pulse
- markedly increased blood pressure.

ADDITIONAL SYMPTOMS OF A RED-BACK SPIDER BITE

- intense local pain which increases and spreads
- small hairs stand on end
- patchy sweating
- headache
- muscle weakness or spasms.

POSSIBLE SIGNS AND SYMPTOMS OF OTHER SPIDER BITES

- burning sensation
- swelling
- blistering.

Management of spider bites

1 Follow **DRABCD**.

2 Lie casualty down.

3 Calm casualty.

4 Apply management for:

Funnel-web/Mouse spider

- apply a firm pressure immobilisation bandage starting just above fingers or toes and as far up limb as possible *(see p. 160)*

- ensure the casualty does not move

- **call 000** for an ambulance.

Red-back

- apply cold pack/compress to area to lessen the pain *(see p. 159)*

- seek medical aid promptly.

Other spiders

- wash with soap and water

- apply cold pack/compress to relieve pain/discomfort

- seek medical aid if casualty develops severe symptoms.

Insect stings

Stings from bees, wasps and ants are always painful. Bee stings are usually left behind in the skin with the venom sac attached and have to be removed, usually with a fingernail. The European wasp can give multiple stings and inject a significant amount of venom.

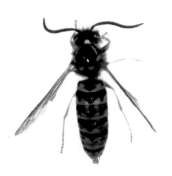

European Wasp

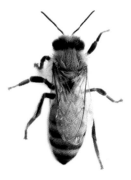

Bee

Fire ants, accidently introduced into Australia in the late 20th century, can cause painful, burning stings with discomfort that may last for an hour or more. The painful red stung area changes into an itchy blister or pustule (pus-filled sac) over the following days. This itchy or painful blister may remain up to a week. Fire ant stings, like those from bees and wasps, can also result in acute severe allergic reactions.

Ticks are very small, but after feeding on the casualty's blood, the abdomen of the female tick becomes engorged and may be up to 1 cm across. They attach themselves to the body and may be found in body crevices and hairy areas. Their bite is painless and the casualty may not be aware that he or she is carrying a tick. If the tick is attached for several days, the venom of the Australian paralysis tick (or scrub tick) can cause serious symptoms. The venom of a bush tick may cause paralysis, especially in young children. Many ticks do not cause paralysis but may cause local irritation or a skin nodule. Some people may have an allergic reaction, which may be severe. A variety of ticks can be found throughout Australia; however, paralysis ticks occur mainly along coastal eastern Australia from Queensland to northern Tasmania.

SIGNS AND SYMPTOMS OF BITES AND STINGS

- pain at the site—sometimes extreme pain (European wasp)
- swelling and redness
- muscle weakness (tick)
- difficulty in breathing and swallowing (tick)
- itchy and painful blisters.

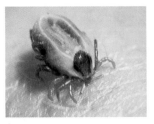

Tick

Management of bites and stings

1 Follow **DRABCD**.

2 Apply cold compress.

3 If severe allergic reaction:

- **call 000** for an ambulance.

- if casualty is carrying medication for an allergic reaction (e.g. EpiPen®), it should be used immediately *(see p. 348)*.

4 Apply specific management for:

Bee sting

- remove sting—scrape sideways with your fingernail or the side of a sharp object (e.g. a knife).

Tick bite

- remove tick—using fine tipped forceps or equivalent, press skin down around the tick's embedded mouth part

- grip the mouth part firmly, lift gently to detach the tick—do not squeeze the body of the tick with fingers or forceps during removal.

5 Apply a cold compress to relieve pain if necessary.

6 Monitor signs of life—give CPR if necessary.

7 Seek medical aid.

Note: If the casualty has a rash, persistent headache, fever, aching joints or a history of allergy, seek medical advice immediately.

Leech bite

- Leeches feed on the blood of humans and other vertebrates. Their bite is painless, but oozes blood due to an anti-clotting substance in leech saliva. Even when removed, the wound may take days to heal. The leech should not be pulled off as this may cause a severe wound. Instead, the leech may be removed by either the application of salt or touching it with a hot object, e.g. an extinguished hot match. Treat the wound as a bleeding injury.

Allergic reaction to a sting

While insect stings can be very painful, they are rarely fatal. They can, however, be dangerous for those who have an allergic reaction. An allergic reaction can happen almost immediately and can result in blockage of the airway—anaphylactic shock *(see p. 309)*.

SIGNS AND SYMPTOMS
- rash, itching
- swollen eyelids, face, or neck tissues
- altered voice (e.g. high-pitched or 'crowing' sound)
- wheezing
- respiratory distress
- altered conscious state.

Management of an allergic reaction caused by a bite or sting

1 Follow **DRABCD**.

2 Apply a pressure immobilisation bandage to the affected limb *(see p. 160)*.

3 At the same time, ask casualty if they are carrying an EpiPen®. If so, where state and territory legislation permits, administer according to instructions on the Anaphylaxis Action Plan recommended by the Australasian Society of Clinical Immunology and Allergy website: www.allergy.org.au *(see p. 309)*.

4 **Call 000** for an ambulance.

5 Ensure the casualty keeps still.

6 If the casualty is conscious:
   • help to a position that assists breathing.

   If casualty is unconscious:
   • Follow **DRABCD**.

Animal bites

All animals (and humans) carry bacteria and other organisms in their mouths. Bites may puncture the skin. Untreated bites are highly likely to become infected.

Management of animal bites

1 Follow **DRABCD**.

2 Control bleeding—use direct pressure and elevation.

3 Apply dressing and bandage firmly.

4 Immobilise if bite on a limb.

5 Seek medical aid.

Bat bite

1 Handling of bats, whether injured or not, MUST be avoided. Their bite can transmit a fatal disease.

2 Anyone either bitten or scratched by a bat should immediately:

• wash the wounds thoroughly with soap water

• promptly seek medical advice regardless of the site or severity of the wound.

Tropical marine bites and stings

Australia's tropical waters contain a number of animals whose stings can be life-threatening. Many beaches in Australia's north have large signs warning of the danger of stingers. Swim only at patrolled mainland beaches in northern Australia during the 'stinger season' in summer, called locally the 'wet season'. The presence of jellyfish and their risk are monitored at patrolled mainland beaches.

Vinegar is the single substance most likely to save a life in the early management for box jellyfish and Irukandji stings and recommended for most other tropical jellyfish stings.

Vinegar is used to manage tropical stings such as:

- known or suspected box jellyfish
- known or suspected Irukandji
- tropical stings of unknown origin.

DO NOT use hot water on tropical marine stings.

Box jellyfish

The box jellyfish has a large, virtually transparent, square shaped body with tentacles draping from each of the four corners of the body. Each tentacle has millions of individual stinging cells called nematocysts, each containing a tiny dose of venom which 'fires' into the skin upon contact. The more tentacles which make skin contact, the larger the venom dose injected. Documented human stings from the box jellyfish extend from Lagrange Bay, south-west of Broome in Western Australia (WA), to Bustard Head, south of Gladstone, Queensland, while confirmed sightings of smaller box jellyfish species extend from Exmouth in WA to northern New South Wales.

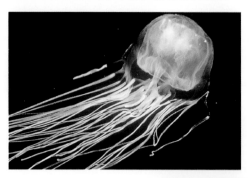

Box jellyfish

(bell 15–25cm, tentacles up to 3 metres)

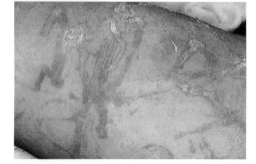

Sting from a box jellyfish

Irukandji jellyfish

Irukandji jellyfish can cause single or mass stinging in tropical Australian waters. The initial sting, while the bather is in the water, is usually trivial. Within 5 to 40 minutes or so, a dramatic collection of signs and symptoms develop. These may include excruciating abdominal and back pains, nausea and vomiting, profuse sweating, increased blood pressure, and a peculiar but distressing feeling of impending doom.

Always consider the possibility of Irukandji stinging if bathers or surfers present with severe pain either in the water of after emerging from the sea. If one person is stung by an Irukandji, be prepared to manage multiple casualties. Warn other bathers that Irukandji jellyfish are in the water; some casualties may need to be helped from the water to prevent drowning.

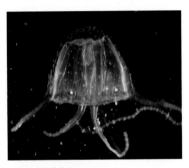

Irukandji jellyfish
(10–11 mm bell height)

Sea anemone

There are two types of sea anemone. One has little envenomation jaws on its surface and the other has long sharp venomous spines which lodge in the flesh and may in some cases may require surgical removal. The stings may cause severe local pain.

Jimble

The jimble is a translucent jellyfish with four tentacles and may be difficult to see in the water. The body is about 2–5 cm in diameter and 3 cm wide with tentacles 6–8 cm long. Jimbles can be found along the entire coastline of Australia and the Pacific area in swarms, normally in warm water at the sea surface at dusk and dawn.

Management of Box Jellyfish, Irukandji, sea anemone, jimble

1   Follow **DRABCD**.

    In rescuing a casualty from the water, don't become enmeshed in tentacles yourself.

2   **Call 000** for an ambulance.

3   Calm casualty; restrain casualty from rubbing stung area.

4   Flood the entire stung area with vinegar for at least 30 seconds to neutralise stinging cells and prevent further envenomation..

Note: DO NOT *wash with fresh water; it will cause additional nematocyst discharge.*

5   If no vinegar is available, flick off any remnants of tentacles with a stick; wash well with **seawater** to remove microscopic stinging cells adhering to skin.

6   Remain with the casualty, if possible, until medical aid arrives.

7   Be prepared to give CPR if necessary.

8   Keep casualty at rest to decrease absorption of the toxin.

Note: After flooding the stung area in vinegar for 30 seconds, applying a cold pack may provide pain relief (do not apply hot water).

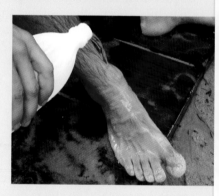

Other non-tropical minor jellyfish stings

Many other species of jellyfish occur in non-tropical Australian coastal waters; some of these may cause severe stings and allergic reactions.

Management of non-tropical minor jellyfish stings

1 Rest and reassure the casualty; restrain casualty from rubbing stung area.

2 Keep the casualty under constant observation.

3 Pick off any adherent tentacles with fingers.

4 Rinse stung area well with seawater to remove invisible stinging cells (DO NOT wash with fresh water).

5 Apply cold packs or wrapped ice for pain relief.

6 If local pain is unrelieved, generalised pain develops or sting area is large (e.g. half of limb) call 000 for an ambulance.

Bluebottle (Pacific Man-O-War)

The bluebottles inhabit waters throughout Australia and often found in swarms. The sting causes immediate pain usually lasting about 30 minutes, with typical oval-shaped blanched wheals and surrounding redness of the skin. The bluebottle, if large (tentacles can be up to 10 m in length) is more dangerous and can produce a severe envenomation syndrome with muscle pains, nausea, vomiting.

Management of bluebottle (Pacific Man-O-War) sting

1 Pick off any adherent tentacles with fingers (this has been shown not to be harmful to the rescuer).

2 Rinse stung area well with seawater to remove invisible stinging cells.

3 Place the casualty's stung area in hot water (no hotter than the rescuer can comfortably tolerate).

4 If local pain is unrelieved by heat, or if hot water is not available, apply a cold pack or wrapped ice for pain relief.

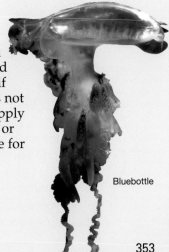

Bluebottle

Blue-ringed octopus bite and cone shell sting

The blue-ringed octopus is found in Australian waters. When provoked, it flashes vivid blue and gold rings on the body and tentacles. Bites usually occur when the octopus is removed from the water and is in contact with exposed skin. The bite may not be painful and a spot of blood on the skin may be the only sign. Not every bite results in envenomation and more often results in tingling around the mouth and mild weakness. In severe cases, paralysis, including respiratory paralysis may develop quickly, threatening life.

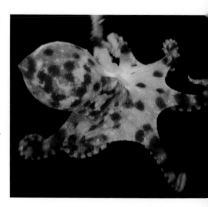

Blue-ringed octopus (up to 20cm)

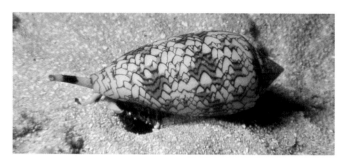

Cone shell

The cone shell is found mostly in tropical waters and warmer temperate sea floors and reefs. Envenomation may occur when the shell is picked up and a barb is fired from the pointed end of the shell causing local pain. The envenomation may cause progressive paralysis, and breathing to cease. Fortunately, cone shell stings are rare.

Management of blue-ringed octopus bite and cone shell stings

1 Follow **DRABCD**.

2 Calm the casualty.

3 Apply pressure immobilisation bandage (*see p. 160*).

4 Splint the bandaged limb.

5 Ensure the casualty does not move.

6 Give CPR if necessary.

7 **Call 000** for an ambulance.

Note: The venom causes muscle paralysis leading to breathing failure and possibly death. Cardiopulmonary resuscitation must be continued until medical aid arrives, because, although paralysis is long lasting, it will eventually abate.

Spines and barbs from creatures such as catfish, stonefish, bullrout and crown-of-thorns starfish

Injuries due to penetration by the spines or barbs from this group of creatures always contain infected and toxic material. Prevention is very important. Protective footwear must always be worn when walking on rocky, muddy, or coral-encrusted reef or intertidal regions. They are always painful. Handling these creatures should be done with particular care.

Management of spine and barb injuries from creatures such as bullrout, catfish, stonefish, crown-of-thorns starfish

1 Follow **DRABCD**.

2 Calm the casualty.

3 If the wound is on a limb, remove any remaining sting barbs; clean visible foreign material from the wound.

4 Place the casualty's stung foot or hand in hot water (as hot as the casualty can comfortably tolerate by testing the water temperature with their other hand or foot).

5 **Call 000** for an ambulance.

Stingray

The stinging mechanism (spine) is attached to the stingray's whip-like tail and may cause significant trauma as well as envenomation. The spine may snap off and become embedded in the wound. The venom is contained in tissues around the barb and is released into the wound as the barb penetrates the casualty's flesh. Immediate intense burning pain, bleeding from the wound and a variety of symptoms may occasionally be experienced, some of which may be serious, such as possible breathing difficulties. Most injuries occur on the lower leg of waders who step on a stingray on the sandy shallow sea floor. All injuries should be referred for medical assessment. Injuries to torso, neck, head, groin or bone, or those which cause severe bleeding, require immediate attention.

Warning

Any stingray injury to the chest, abdomen, neck, head, groin, or bone is a medical emergency. Do not remove embedded stingray spines, especially from these areas.

Management of injuries from a stingray

1   Follow **DRABCD**.

2   Stop any severe bleeding and calm casualty.

3   Do not remove embedded spines.

4   If the casualty is stung on the hand, arm leg or foot, ensure bleeding has stopped before placing stung part in hot water—as hot as the casualty can comfortably tolerate by testing the water temperature with their other foot or hand. Beware of causing burns to the casualty.

5   **Call 000** for an ambulance.

17

Poisoning

The number of deaths in Australia from accidental poisonings has declined in recent years because of education campaigns and the introduction of childproof containers. However, many thousands of accidental poisonings still occur, especially to children, resulting in the loss of lives each year.

Poisons can be ingested, inhaled, absorbed or injected into the body. Most people are aware that Australia has a number of lethal venomous snakes and spiders. Poisonous fumes can be inhaled from a car exhaust. Most people are aware that many household substances—cleaning products, pesticides, alcohol and medication—are potentially dangerous poisons, particularly for children.

Poisoning

Many substances in the home or workplace are poisonous. Many containers display a poisons symbol to indicate the danger. Many do not. A poison is any substance which causes harm to body tissues. A toxin is a poison made by a living organism (e.g. plant, animal or micro-organism). A venom is a toxin which is injected by a fang or sting (e.g. from a spider, snake or fish).

Tobacco, alcohol, some common plants, solvents, contaminated food, detergents, glues, adhesives, aerosols can be poisonous. A common form of poisoning results from improperly using medications. Many substances not harmful in small amounts can be poisonous in large amounts.

All households contain solvents and petroleum products which, if swallowed, may cause severe lung or organ damage. Caustic substances such as oven or drain cleaners and dishwasher powder or liquids may, if swallowed, may cause serious internal injury and burns.

Poisoning may occur in the workplace particularly when new and dangerous chemicals are introduced in process work or manufacturing, or when routine is unexpectedly broken.

Poisoning may be accidental or intentional, the latter usually in the context of a suicide attempt. Fortunately, deaths from accidental poisoning are rare in Australia. The use of childproof containers and single-dose 'bubble packaging' of tablets has meant that child fatalities from accidental poisoning are very uncommon. Occasionally, adults who are using novel chemicals in newly-acquired hobbies are poisoned because of their unfamiliarity with such agents as glues, solvents and fuels.

POISONS INFORMATION CENTRES

Poisons Information Centres exist in every State and Territory. The national number for information about poisons, and help in an emergency, is:

13 11 26

How poisons enter the body

Poisons can enter the body through the mouth (ingested/swallowed), nose (inhaled/breathed in) or through the skin (absorbed/injected). Once a poison has entered the bloodstream, it is transported swiftly to all parts of the body.

HOW POISONS ENTER THE BODY

Absorbed through eyes (e.g. chemicals).

Inhaled—gases, solvents, vapours, fumes.

Ingested (swallowed) through digestive tract walls.

Injected—drugs (e.g. narcotics), venoms from snakes, fish, insects, spiders—can be absorbed into the circulation very quickly.

Absorbed through the skin—corrosives, pesticides, other strong chemicals.

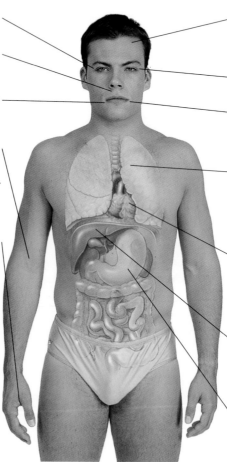

HOW POISONS AFFECT THE BODY

Brain—poisons can cause confusion, delirium, seizures, unconsciousness.

Eyes—can cause burns and irritation, scarring.

Lips, mouth, oesophagus—swallowed poisons can burn.

Respiratory tract—respiratory distress, poisons causing unconsciousness can slow breathing and cause airway blockage.

Heart—some poisons interfere with functioning (e.g. anti-depressant drug overdose, oleander poisoning).

Liver, kidneys—can be seriously damaged by overload of toxins (e.g. paracetamol overdose, mushrooms).

Digestive system—poisons can cause vomiting, abdominal pain, diarrhoea.

Blood—poisons can prevent red cells carrying oxygen to tissues (e.g. carbon monoxide, cyanide).

Ingested poisons

Commonly ingested poisons include contaminated or poisonous food (e.g. some mushrooms), substances such as alcohol, medication (e.g. paracetamol, sleeping tablets—if taken in excess of normal dosage), household items (e.g. cleaners, dishwashing powders, kerosene, pesticides) and some plants (e.g. oleander).

Food-related illness is usually associated with poor hygiene and food handling practices. It results from eating food contaminated by bacteria or by toxins produced by bacteria in the food usually resulting from inappropriate storage or spoiling. Bacterial food poisoning is often caused by *Salmonella* germs or by toxins from *Staphylococcus* germs.

Drinking large quantities of alcohol affect people in different ways and can result in poisoning. Alcohol depresses the activity of the nervous system which can result in severe impairment of physical and mental abilities. Unconsciousness can follow, breathing may be impaired and vomit may be inhaled, blocking the airway.

Common household poisons

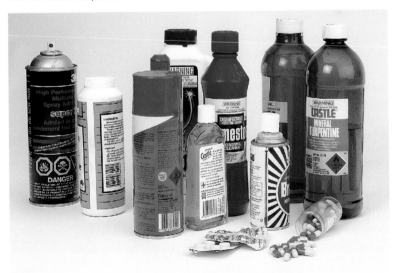

Inhaled poisons

Poisoning by inhalation occurs when a person breathes toxic fumes from a gas or burning solids or liquids. Besides causing breathing problems such fumes can result in headaches, nausea and dizziness. Inhaled fumes may affect the person's consciousness. Inhaled poisons include the fumes of carbon monoxide (e.g. emitted by car engine exhausts or defective heating equipment), and gases such as methane (e.g. in mines, wells, sewers), chlorine (e.g. in cleaning products or swimming pool chemicals) and fumes (from paints, glues and industrial chemicals).

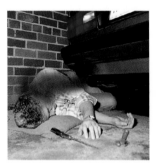

Warning

Anyone who is unconscious after inhaling poisonous gas or fumes should be taken into a safe, fresh air environment immediately. High-flow oxygen is urgently needed under these circumstances.

Absorbed poisons

Absorbed poisons enter the body through the skin or mucous membranes. These poisons include dry and wet chemicals, fertilisers, pesticides and any other substance that causes irritation and reddening of the skin at the point of contact. Contact with water makes some dry chemicals (e.g. dishwashing crystals) more caustic. Copious amounts of running water are used to flood the exposed area of skin. Repeated rinsing of the mouth can help but the water should be spat out rather than swallowed. Poisons splashed into the eye can also be absorbed. Flush the eye with gentle running water for 20 minutes.

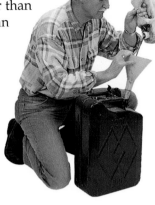

Injected poisons

Injected poisons may enter the body as a result of a bite or sting from a spider, marine animal, fish, snake or insect. Drugs injected with a needle cause many accidental and suicidal deaths each year.

SIGNS AND SYMPTOMS

The signs and symptoms of poisoning depend on the nature of the substance and, in some cases, how it entered the body. Any of the following may be observed:

- bite or injection marks, with or without local swelling
- contamination of skin
- burns around and inside mouth or on tongue
- smell of fumes
- odours on breath
- burning pain from mouth through to stomach
- nausea and/or vomiting
- abdominal pain
- change of skin colour—blueness around lips
- difficulty breathing

- tight feeling in chest
- drowsiness
- headache
- ringing in ears
- blurred vision
- sudden collapse
- seizures (convulsions).

Remember

1 Record the names of the chemicals, solvents or poisons involved.
2 Contact the Poisons Information Centre 13 11 26 for specific advice on management.
3 Send any containers and/or suicide notes with casualty to hospital.
4 Send any vomit with casualty to hospital.

General and specific management of poisoning

Management of poisoning—general

Unconscious casualty

1 Follow **DRABCD**—remove yourself and the casualty from any danger.

2 **Call 000** for an ambulance.

3 Call fire services if atmosphere is contaminated with smoke or gas.

Note: For drug and alcohol poisoning in children see page 436.

Conscious casualty

1 Check for danger—remove yourself and the casualty from any danger.

2 Listen to casualty—give reassurance.

3 Determine nature of substance, if possible, and record.

4 **Call 000** for an ambulance.

5 Call Poisons Information Centre—13 11 26.

Management of poisoning—specific

Ingested poisons

For all ingested poisons, including a corrosive, petroleum-based, medicinal, or unknown substance:

1 Do not induce vomiting.

2 Do not give anything by mouth.

3 Wash corrosive substance off mouth and face with water, or wipe off.

Inhaled poisons

1 Move the casualty and yourself to fresh air.

2 Loosen tight clothing.

3 Consider using oxygen therapy is necessary.

Absorbed poisons

1 Protect yourself (if possible) by wearing disposable gloves, goggles and protective clothing.

2 Ask the casualty to remove contaminated clothing and place the contaminated clothes in a plastic bag—be careful to avoid contact with your own skin.

3 Flush the casualty's skin with large amounts of running water.

Capsicum spray exposure

Capsicum spray is available in a number of commercial forms and is being used more commonly by police forces all over Australia to subdue aggressive people. It is carried in a spray can and is regarded as an offensive weapon. When used as a weapon, the spray is aimed at the face. The active agent can be absorbed by the mouth, nose, and eyes and across intact skin without damage to tissue. While it is intended that only the aggressor will be incapacitated, police, bystanders and first aiders can also be affected.

Exposure to capsicum spray causes intense pain, spasm of the eyelids and a wheeze (often worse in a person prone to asthma). These symptoms will incapacitate most people exposed to the spray.

Management of casualty sprayed with capsicum

1 Follow **DRABCD**.

2 Protect your body, hands and eyes as much as possible using goggles, gloves and clothing.

3 Absorb excess capsicum solution with paper towel or similar and dispose of thoughtfully.

4 Follow police directions, if such are indicated.

5 If casualty is cooperative, move to fresh air and place in a comfortable sitting position. If this is not possible, ventilate the room.

6 Check airway and breathing—if necessary, give oxygen at a rate of 8–15 litre per minute.

7 If casualty has breathing difficulty, use reliever puffer—as for management of asthma *(see p. 314).*

8 Wash exposed areas with copious quantities of cool tap water.

9 Wash eyes with water at room temperature for at least 15 minutes.

10 If affected area is below neck, an ice pack may be applied for 15 minutes to give relief.

11 Seek medical aid.

Note: The person may still be agitated and uncontrolled. There may also be excess spray on the casualty, their handlers, in the air and room and on flat surfaces, floor or ground. Ensure that police are still close by and you have a secure escape route or 'back away' area, if attacked.

18

Exposure to heat and cold

One tenth of Australia has significant periods of below-freezing weather, and most of the continent has extensive periods of extreme heat. Australians travel overseas to areas where they may experience extremes of temperature. Exposure to these extremes of heat or cold may cause suffering, injury, and even death.

These situations are not confined to the outback or snowfields. The casualty may be the elderly person sitting quietly in a cold room, the homeless teenager wandering the streets, the victim of a boating mishap, the lost bushwalker or even the person exercising in the middle of a hot summer's day.

This chapter discusses what first aid can be given to casualties suffering from conditions caused by heat and cold, and also focuses on prevention.

Exposure to heat and cold

The body works efficiently only as long as it remains at a constant temperature. If the body's temperature drops more than a few degrees below the normal of approximately 37°C, or rises significantly, it cannot function properly.

Maintaining normal body temperature

The body is like a house with an efficient ducted heating and cooling system. It maintains a constant temperature by balancing heat production and heat loss.

Sources of heat

Eating provides the body with fuel to burn. The conversion
of food into energy (the process of metabolism) provides much
of the body's heat, as does muscular activity such as exercising
or shivering. Heat is also absorbed from outside sources such
as the sun, hot air or hot food.

Cooling

The circulatory system provides the ducting system. When the
body needs to lose heat, blood vessels near the surface of the
skin widen (dilate) to allow more warm blood to be brought to
the skin's surface for heat to escape. The evaporation of sweat
from the skin's surface also causes heat loss. Moving air—from
a fan or a breeze—speeds up the cooling process. The faster the
air moves, the quicker sweat evaporates and the layer of
warmed air around the body is swept away.

Conserving heat

If the body needs to conserve heat, blood vessels near the skin's surface get smaller (constrict) to keep heat inside. The skin looks pale or white and feels cold. Sweating stops and muscles contract, causing goose bumps which raise hairs on the body in an attempt to 'trap' warm air at the skin's surface.

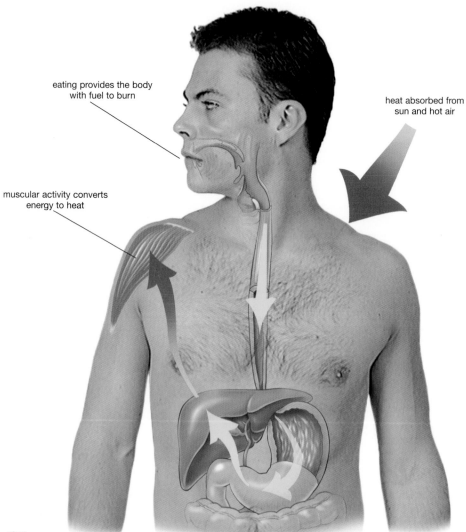

eating provides the body with fuel to burn

heat absorbed from sun and hot air

muscular activity converts energy to heat

The hot environment

People are at risk of heat illness in humid or hot climates. Someone working in a hot environment, such as a boiler room, is at risk because the air heats the body at a rate faster than it can cool itself.

In a hot, dry climate, evaporation is very fast; therefore the body can adapt to the higher temperatures. In a humid climate, evaporation is slower. Therefore it can be more difficult to maintain core body temperature in Cairns when it is 25°C and humid than in Bourke at a dry 35°C.

The importance of water

Heat can interfere with the body's water balance. The body needs a minimum amount of water to carry out normal functions such as blood circulation and excretion of waste. For healthy adults in non-active, cool conditions, a minimum water intake of about 1.7 litres is needed each day. In hot climates, where physical work is being undertaken in the open, an intake of up to 15 litres each day may be required.

Heavy sweating removes water and salts from the body at a faster rate than normal. Total blood volume decreases because there is less fluid available for the plasma. More salt and water are retained by the kidneys. Collection of urine in the bladder is slower, with a higher concentration of waste products causing urine to be a darker yellow colour. This is a warning sign that plasma volume is falling. If this is not corrected, the body becomes dehydrated.

People do not always realise that they are not replacing fluid lost through sweating. They may not feel thirsty—or thirsty enough—to realise the importance of drinking more water. Because of this, troops on training exercises and people in fun runs or working out at gyms are taught and encouraged to drink water at regular intervals.

When moving to a hot climate a person's daily intake of water needs to increase. Body salts may also be depleted, so extra salt may be needed in food. If water is replaced but not body salts, the concentration of salt will be too low, impairing normal functioning.

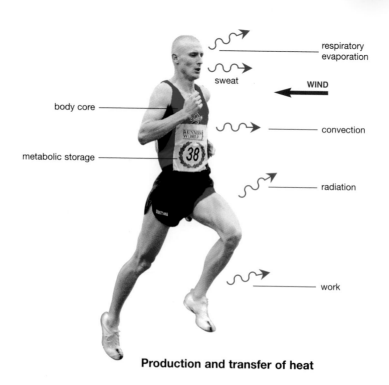

solar
radiation

respiratory
evaporation

sweat

WIND

body core

convection

metabolic storage

radiation

work

Production and transfer of heat

Heat-induced conditions

Physical activity, particularly in hot conditions, may cause the body to become overheated. This can result in heat-induced swelling—feet and hands swell in warm weather.

Management of heat-induced swelling

1 Raise the casualty's legs.

2 Encourage the casualty to gently exercise.

3 Keep casualty cool.

Heat cramps are a result of losing too much water and salt through sweating causing painful muscle cramps, usually in legs and abdomen.

Management of muscle cramps

1 Ask the casualty to stop the activity and rest in a cool environment.

2 Gently stretch the affected muscle.

3 Apply an ice pack.

4 Give cool water to drink.

In addition to swelling and cramps, more serious heat-induced conditions can also develop.

Heat exhaustion

Heat exhaustion results from being physically active in a hot environment without taking the right precautions. It can affect athletes, workers who must wear heavy clothing (e.g. firefighters, factory workers), the young, the elderly who compensate poorly for heat, those wearing unsuitable clothing on a hot day, and people suffering from dehydration.

Fluid loss through sweating reduces the amount of water in the body so that the blood volume falls. Increasing blood flow to the skin makes the blood volume even less effective, reducing blood flow to vital organs. As the circulatory system is affected, the body goes into a mild form of shock.

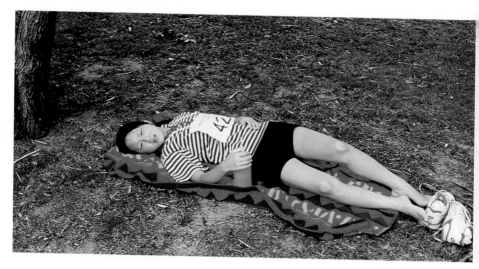

SIGNS AND SYMPTOMS

- feeling hot, exhausted, weak and fatigued
- persistent headache
- thirst and nausea
- giddiness and faintness
- rapid breathing and shortness of breath
- pale, cool, clammy skin
- rapid, weak pulse.

Management of heat exhaustion

1 Move the casualty to lie down in a cool place with circulating air.

2 Loosen tight clothing and remove unnecessary garments.

3 Sponge with cold water.

4 Give cool water to drink if conscious.

5 Seek medical aid if casualty vomits or does not recover promptly.

Heatstroke

Heatstroke is a potentially lethal condition. Water levels in the body become so low that sweating stops and body temperature rises because the body can no longer cool itself. The brain and other vital organs, such as the kidneys and heart, begin to fail.

Those most at risk of heatstroke include infants left in closed cars on a warm to hot day, athletes attempting to run long distances in hot weather, unfit workers, overweight alcoholics in hot climates, the elderly and the sick.

SIGNS AND SYMPTOMS

- high body temperature of 40°C or more
- flushed, dry skin
- initially a pounding, rapid pulse which gradually weakens
- headache, nausea and/or vomiting
- dizziness and visual disturbances
- irritability and mental confusion
- altered mental state which may progress to seizures and unconsciousness.

Management of heatstroke

1 Follow **DRABCD**.

2 Remove the casualty to a cool place.

3 Remove almost all clothing; loosen anything tight.

4 Apply cold packs or ice to areas of large blood vessels (neck, groin and armpits) to accelerate cooling.

5 If possible, cover body with a wet sheet; fan to increase air circulation (stop cooling when body feels cold to the touch).

6 **Call 000** for an ambulance.

7 If casualty is fully conscious and is able to swallow, give fluids.

Note: This casualty needs urgent medical aid.

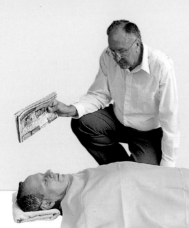

The cold environment

Maintaining body temperature

Just as the body reacts to external heat conditions, it also reacts to cold. To conserve body heat, blood vessels in the skin shut down to prevent the body's 'core heat' escaping. This will affect extremities (fingers and toes) before other exposed areas of the body.

Wind and skin wetness increases the effects of cold air. Wind speed and air temperature combine to give the 'windchill factor'. Clothing, food and water intake, and physical exercise can also affect body cooling.

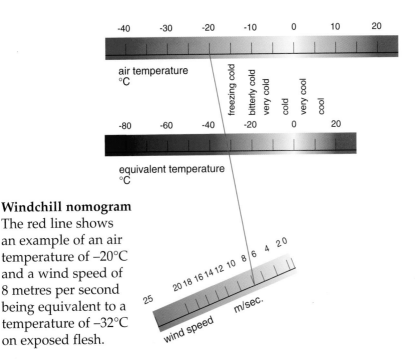

Windchill nomogram
The red line shows an example of an air temperature of –20°C and a wind speed of 8 metres per second being equivalent to a temperature of –32°C on exposed flesh.

How the body loses heat

Heat may be lost by:

- **radiation**—heat radiates from the body, especially from the head

- **evaporation**—the body produces sweat which evaporates from the skin's surface to keep the body cool on a hot day

- **breathing**—cold air is inhaled, warmed and humidified by the body, and exhaled. The moisture in exhaled air on a cold day condenses into a misty breath

- **conduction**—when you sit on or touch a cold object, heat flows directly from the body to the cold surface (e.g. sitting on a cold chair or the cold ground)

- **convection**—the thin layer of air on the surface of the skin rises and is replaced by cooler air, causing heat loss, even in the absence of wind or movement.

How the body loses heat

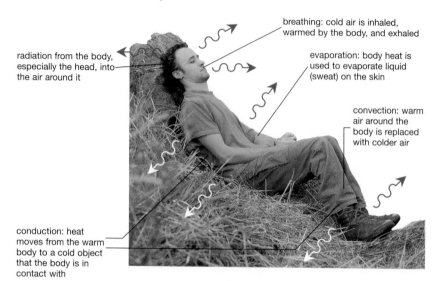

breathing: cold air is inhaled, warmed by the body, and exhaled

radiation from the body, especially the head, into the air around it

evaporation: body heat is used to evaporate liquid (sweat) on the skin

convection: warm air around the body is replaced with colder air

conduction: heat moves from the warm body to a cold object that the body is in contact with

Humans are able to adjust to the cold in a number of ways.

Decreasing heat loss

- Exposure to cold conditions causes blood vessels near skin surface to constrict, thereby reducing the amount of heat radiated away.

- Use of clothing and shelter insulates the body from cold and wind.

- Use of artificial heating warms the surroundings—decreasing the difference between ambient and body temperatures.

Increasing heat production

- Exercise causes metabolic heat production to increase considerably.

- Shivering is a form of involuntary exercise which occurs as the core temperature starts to drop.

People most at risk

Anyone can suffer cold-induced conditions related to over-exposure. Some groups are particularly prone. They include:

- the elderly—often have poor circulation, reduced body insulation and low metabolic rate
- babies and young children—lose body heat quickly, especially from the head
- people already weakened through lack of food, fatigue or injury
- people under the influence of alcohol or other drugs—more because of effect on behaviour than any possible alcohol-induced dilation of the blood vessels
- people with certain health problems (e.g. thyroid and pituitary disorders, certain skin conditions), stroke, trauma, burns, starvation, those confined to bed or a wheelchair and those taking certain medication—especially some psychiatric drugs; anyone who is trapped or immobilised.

Cold-induced conditions

SIGNS AND SYMPTOMS

When the body temperature falls, early warning signs may include:

- . feeling cold
- shivering
- clumsiness and slurred speech
- apathy and irrational behaviour.

As the body temperature continues to drop:

- shivering usually ceases
- pulse may be difficult to find
- heart rate may slow
- level of consciousness continues to decline.

At around 30°C body temperature:

- unconsciousness is likely
- heart rhythm is increasingly likely to change.

As the body temperature falls further the heart may arrest, resulting in death.

Hypothermia

Hypothermia occurs when the body's warming mechanisms fail, or are overwhelmed, and body temperature drops below 35°C. Hypothermia has the potential to develop into a serious condition if not recognised and treated at an early stage.

Sometimes hypothermia is mistaken for other conditions such as drunkenness, a stroke or drug abuse. This is especially so in a city where it might be assumed that conditions would be unlikely to cause hypothermia.

Management of hypothermia

1 Follow **DRABCD**.

2 Remove the casualty to a warm, dry place.

3 Protect casualty and yourself from wind, rain, sleet, cold, and wet ground.

4 Handle the casualty as gently as possible.

5 Avoid excess activity or movement.

6 Maintain the casualty in a horizontal position.

7 Remove wet clothing.

8 Place casualty between blankets or in sleeping bag, and wrap in a space blanket * or similar.

9 Cover the head to maintain body heat.

10 Give casualty warm drinks if conscious (but not alcohol).

11 Provide warmth to the casualty:

- direct body-to-body contact may be the only means of rewarming available; however, this method is fairly ineffective and may even interfere with casualty's spontaneous rewarming by shivering

- hot water bottles, heat packs and other sources of external heating may be applied to casualty's neck, armpits and groin, but caution must be taken to avoid burns; aim to stabilise core temperature rather than attempt rapid rewarming.

12 If hypothermia is severe, **call 000** for an ambulance.

13 Remain with the casualty until medical aid arrives.

Note: Although a space blanket reflects radiated heat back to the body, it can also conduct heat away unless some form of insulation such as blankets, sleeping mat, even thick layers of newspaper is provided, either inside or outside the space blanket.

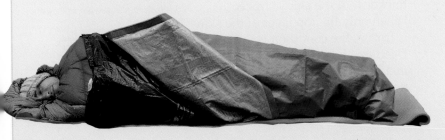

Always consider the possibility of hypothermia if the weather is cold and wet or windy, and especially if all three conditions apply following immersion to those inadequately clothed; and to 'at risk' groups such as infants or the elderly.

Babies may also become hypothermic in rooms which would not pose a threat to an adult. Babies lose heat very easily. A baby may look healthy, the only signs of hypothermia being cold skin and that the baby is unusually quiet and drowsy or refuses food.

Cautions in first aid for hypothermia

- Pulse may be difficult to find—check with a warm hand for 30 to 45 seconds.
- If casualty starts to shiver, take measures to prevent further heat loss.
- DO NOT rub affected area.
- DO NOT use radiant heat such as fire or electric heaters.
- DO NOT give alcohol.

Note: It is best not to put casualty in a hot bath, as monitoring and/or resuscitation, if needed, may be difficult.

Frostbite

Frostbite occurs when the skin and underlying tissues become frozen as a result of exposure to below zero temperatures. It is a progressive injury. In superficial frostbite the skin can still be moved in relation to the underlying tissue. The full thickness of the skin is frozen. When only the top layer of the skin

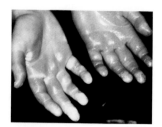

Frostbitten fingers before thawing

is frozen, the condition is sometimes referred to as frostnip. Deep frostbite is recognisable by the skin no longer being mobile in relation to the underlying tissue. The skin and the tissues underneath the skin are frozen, sometimes to the bone.

Stages of frostbite

Stage	Description	Signs and symptoms
Superficial frostbite	The full thickness of the skin is frozen. If only the top layer of the skin is frozen, it is usually called frostnip.	• white, waxy-looking skin • skin is firm to touch, but tissue underneath is soft • may feel pain at first, followed by numbness
Deep frostbite	The skin, and the tissues underneath the skin, are frozen, sometimes to the bone. This is a serious condition, often involving an entire hand.	• white, waxy-looking skin that turns greyish-blue as frostbite progresses • skin feels cold and hard • there is no feeling in the area or foot.

DO NOT rub or massage the frozen area—the tiny ice crystals in the tissues may cause more tissue damage.

DO NOT rewarm with radiant heat (fire, exhaust pipes)—this may rewarm too quickly.

DO NOT apply snow or cold water to area—this may cause further freezing and tissue damage.

DO NOT give person alcohol.

Management of superficial frostbite

1 Follow **DRABCD**.

2 Remove the casualty to a warm, dry place.

3 Rewarm the frostbitten part with body heat—place frostbitten fingers in armpit; place warm hands over frostbitten ears.

4 Prevent affected areas from freezing by ensuring that casualty stops the activity or dresses more appropriately.

Management of deep frostbite

1 Follow **DRABCD**.

2 Prevent further heat loss from the frozen part and the rest of the body.

3 Handle the frozen tissue very gently to prevent further tissue damage.

4 DO NOT rub the arms and legs; keep the casualty as still as possible.

5 Remove casualty to a warm, dry place—if the feet or legs are frozen, don't let the casualty walk.

6 **Call 000** for an ambulance.

If medical help is not readily available, thaw the frozen part as follows:

1 Make the casualty warm and as comfortable as possible.

2 Gently remove the clothing from affected part.

3 Fill a container, large enough to hold the entire frozen part, with warm water—about 40°C; feels warm to the elbow.

4 Remove any jewellery and put the whole frozen part in the water.

5 Keep adding warm water to maintain a constant temperature.

6 Keep the part in the water until it is pink or does not improve any more—this can take up to 40 minutes, and may be painful.

7 Keep the part elevated and warm—do not break any blisters that form.

8 **Call 000** for an ambulance.

Cryogenic burn

A cryogenic burn occurs when the skin touches and sticks to an extremely cold surface such as metal or ice, or comes into contact with liquefied gases, resulting in frostbite. Wearing gloves can prevent this.

Management of cryogenic burn

1 Pour warm water over the part to free it.

2 When free, treat as for superficial frostbite.

3 Seek medical aid for blistering or other tissue damage.

Lifting and moving casualties

Moving a casualty from an accident scene poses dangers for the first aider and for the casualty. Whenever possible, a first aider should always try to give first aid where the casualty is found, as moving can result in further injury or make existing injuries worse.

However, there may be dangers such as an explosion, collapsing structure, traffic hazards, fire or poisonous fumes, or it may not be possible to give first aid due to the casualty's position. A casualty should only be moved if there is immediate danger.

If it is necessary to move a casualty, use a method that poses the least amount of risk to yourself and the casualty. This chapter outlines the ways in which a casualty can be moved with maximum safety.

Moving a casualty

When it is necessary to move a casualty, do so by the quickest and safest means available. Then, while waiting for medical aid to arrive, make sure:

- there is no further danger
- the casualty has a clear airway and is able to breathe
- the most experienced first aider manages the airway (if casualty is unconscious) or the injured part
- bleeding is controlled.

If injuries are serious, it is best to transport the casualty to hospital by ambulance, as improvised transport may reduce the chances of survival. However, an ambulance may not be available.

Before moving the casualty, consider:

- whether you can handle the size and weight of the person without injury to either of you
- what other help is available
- type and seriousness of injuries

- terrain to be crossed
- distance casualty has to be moved
- whether a neck stabilising collar should be applied before movement
- travel or motion sickness which may make casualty worse.

Lifting a casualty

If you need to lift a casualty, it is important to use correct lift techniques to ensure that you and the casualty do not sustain an injury.

When lifting, remember to:

- bend at the knees
- keep your back straight and head up
- keep in a balanced position
- keep your centre of gravity low
- hold the weight close to your body for stability
- take small steps
- work as a team—someone must take role of leader.

Lifting a casualty—general management

Conscious casualty

1 Follow **DRABCD**.

2 Manage all injuries and immobilise fractures.

3 Explain to casualty what you are intending to do.

4 Seek the casualty's help and cooperation.

5 Make sure the casualty feels secure.

6 Always use help to lift—if available.

7 Hold the casualty firmly.

8 Avoid risks where possible.

Moving a casualty with assistance

Two-person human crutch

The two-person human crutch is used to assist a casualty who can support weight on one leg, without making the injury worse and who may also be able to take some weight on the other leg.

Using a two-person human crutch to assist a casualty to walk

1   Help the casualty to stand.

2   Stand one each side of the casualty.

3   First aiders place casualty's arms around their shoulders and hold wrists.

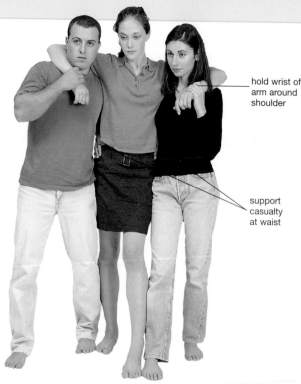

hold wrist of arm around shoulder

support casualty at waist

Two-handed, three-handed and four-handed seats

These lifting techniques are mainly used when the casualty's injuries do not permit the use of the two-person human crutch.

For each hand seat, both first aiders will need to:

1   Hold each other's wrists firmly (left to right; right to left).
2   Squat down to allow casualty to sit on hands.
3   Rise together to lift casualty.
4   Step off on inside foot together.
5   Use crossover step to walk.

Remember

The higher the casualty is lifted the easier carrying will be. Do not have your arms straight when placed under the casualty's thighs, as this makes carrying more difficult. The first aider should, prior to performing these lifts, consider the risk of injury to self and to casualty.

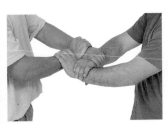

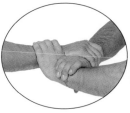
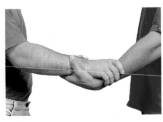

Four-handed seat   Three-handed seat   Two-handed seat

Lifting a casualty using the two-handed seat

The two-handed seat is used for any conscious casualty who can be carried in a seated position, but needs support from both first aiders.

nearest arm is placed around casualty's waist

place other arm under casualty's thighs approximately midway along leg

Two-handed seat

Lifting a casualty using the four-handed seat

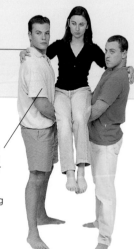

The four-handed seat is used when the casualty is able to use one or both arms to help.

casualty places arms around shoulders

first aiders place arms with hands clasped together under casualty's thighs about midway along leg

Four-handed seat

Fore and aft lift

The fore and aft lift may need to be used when moving a casualty in a narrow area where there is not enough room to use a hand seat.

Lifting a casualty using the fore and aft method

1 Both first aiders bend at the knees, backs as straight as possible, and take hold of the casualty.

2 Casualty's head and shoulders are raised before grasping from behind.

3 First aiders rise together and walk in step.

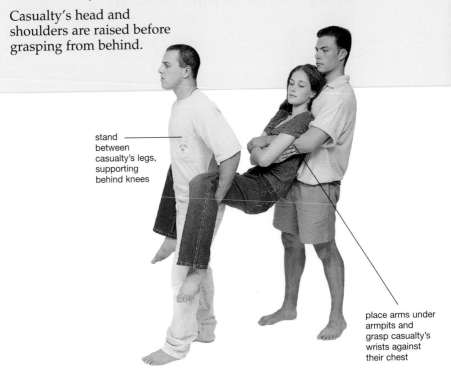

stand between casualty's legs, supporting behind knees

place arms under armpits and grasp casualty's wrists against their chest

Moving a casualty without assistance

The cradle

The cradle is used to carry a child or light casualty. Small children when unconscious are best carried with one arm under the knees and other arm around and supporting the neck—this gives control of the head and allows it to be lowered for drainage of vomit or saliva. Depending on the child's size, the first aider uses either hand to steady the child's crossed arms on chest or abdomen.

Moving a child or light casualty

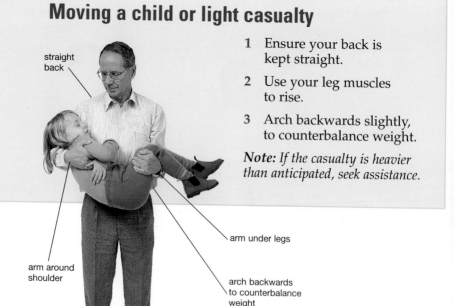

straight back

1 Ensure your back is kept straight.

2 Use your leg muscles to rise.

3 Arch backwards slightly, to counterbalance weight.

Note: If the casualty is heavier than anticipated, seek assistance.

arm under legs

arm around shoulder

arch backwards to counterbalance weight

The human crutch

The human crutch is used when a casualty has an injured leg or foot but is able to walk on the uninjured leg with your assistance—the casualty may also be able to take some weight on the injured leg.

Assisting a casualty to walk

1 Help casualty to stand.

2 Place yourself on casualty's injured side.

3 Take weight of casualty's injured side on your shoulders.

4 Step off together, leading with your inside foot.

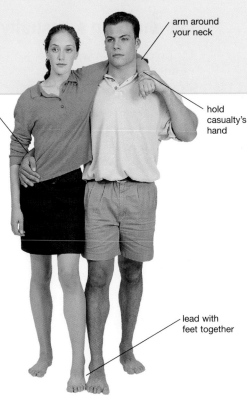

arm around your neck

hold casualty's hand

your nearer arm behind

lead with feet together

Lift and drag

The lift and drag may be used to drag a heavy, helpless casualty from danger.

Warning

Never take the casualty's weight solely on your neck, as this may cause an injury.

Lift and drag a casualty

1 Tie casualty's wrists together.

2 With casualty on back, kneel astride them.

3 Place your head and one arm through casualty's arms.

4 Crawl on hands and knees, lifting casualty's head and shoulders clear of ground.

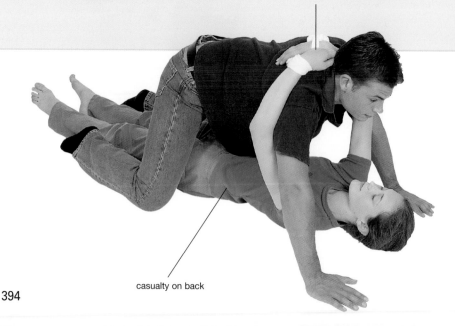

weight distributed across your shoulders and back

casualty on back

Clothes drag

A move is successful if it is carried out without injuring yourself and without causing further injury to the casualty. Using the clothes drag technique to move a casualty will depend on the circumstances and whether there is anyone to help.

A casualty who is conscious and not seriously injured may be able to walk away from the danger with your help. However, if the casualty is unconscious or seriously injured (e.g. fractures or, suspected head or spinal injury), and the situation is such that the casualty must be urgently moved from danger, the clothes drag may be the best technique to use.

Warning

The clothes drag technique may result in back strain for the first aider. Remember to care for your own back safety by using good lifting techniques *(see p. 387)*.

Moving a casualty in an emergency using clothes drag

1 Check for danger—for your safety.

2 If possible, apply a cervical or improvised collar.

3 With casualty on the back, open top buttons of shirt or jacket.

4 Grasp the casualty's cloths behind the neck.

5 Support the casualty's head with their clothing and your forearms.

6 Drag the casualty to safety being careful not to strain your back.

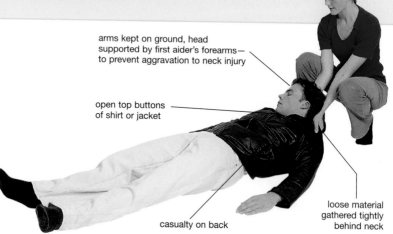

arms kept on ground, head supported by first aider's forearms— to prevent aggravation to neck injury

open top buttons of shirt or jacket

casualty on back

loose material gathered tightly behind neck

Stretchers

Using a stretcher is the safest way to move those who are seriously injured as the chance of further injury is reduced. If moving the casualty is likely to cause any adverse effects, do not move. Wait until an ambulance arrives.

When possible use bystanders to assist with the lift. This shares the load, reduces risk of damage to any lifter and avoids twisting with heavy loads. It is also much more comfortable for the casualty.

The first aider should organise and take charge of the lift. The first aider should also be responsible for an unconscious casualty's head and airway, or for the injured part if the casualty is conscious.

If four people share the lift of a 60 kg casualty (an average weight for a woman), each will only lift 15 kg. The actual lift should be directed by the first aider, giving the instruction that on the command 'lift', all will lift.

It is important to:

- test stretcher for strength and security
- keep stretcher as level as possible
- keep movement to necessary minimum
- correctly position casualty on the stretcher—depending on injuries and condition
- fasten casualty securely to stretcher
- protect the casualty from weather when necessary.

If the casualty has a head injury, is unconscious, or is likely to vomit, place in recovery position on stretcher. Work as quickly and carefully as possible, to ensure safety.

If the casualty has a suspected spinal injury or is unconscious:

- avoid putting pressure on localised areas
- use padding (e.g. sandbags, clothing or blankets) to keep head in a stable position
- DO NOT allow the neck or spine to move or be twisted; use cervical collar or improvise
- remove items such as coins and keys from casualty's pockets.

Securing casualty to a stretcher

When securing casualty to a stretcher, make sure the bandages do not aggravate injuries.

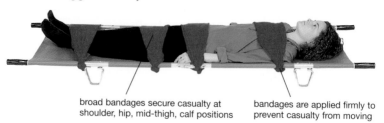

broad bandages secure casualty at shoulder, hip, mid-thigh, calf positions

bandages are applied firmly to prevent casualty from moving

Blanketing a stretcher

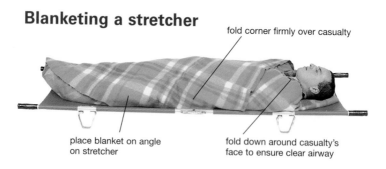

fold corner firmly over casualty

place blanket on angle on stretcher

fold down around casualty's face to ensure clear airway

Loading stretcher without using blankets

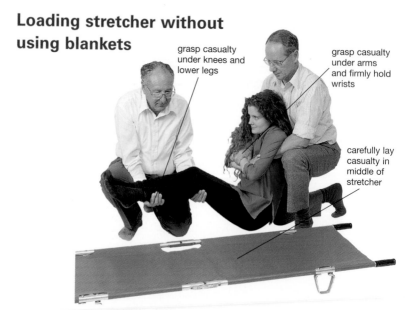

grasp casualty under knees and lower legs

grasp casualty under arms and firmly hold wrists

carefully lay casualty in middle of stretcher

The scoop stretcher

The scoop stretcher is a lifting device that should be removed when the casualty is placed on a standard stretcher, trolley or bed. The stretcher enfolds and closes shut underneath a casualty in the position in which they were found.

The stretcher:

- minimises possibility of complicating injuries
- is adjustable to casualty's physique
- can be manoeuvred through a narrow space
- can be lifted and carried by two or more first aiders.

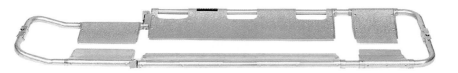

In difficult manoeuvring situations, the casualty should be strapped to the stretcher. A special velcro strap is used to immobilise the head and neck. Take care to:

- avoid pressure on localised areas
- use padding
- remove coins, keys etc. from casualty's pockets
- use sandbags or similar padding to maintain head in a stable position (use cervical collar if available)
- lift stretcher from sides if casualty is heavy
- ensure the casualty is on back and the head is supported so that you can monitor the airway closely.

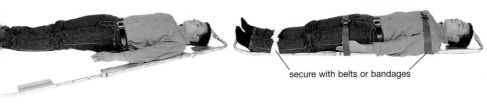

secure with belts or bandages

Blanket lift

A simple blanket can make an excellent lifting device. However, this lift is not used for those whom you suspect to have a neck or spinal injury.

Lifting and loading a casualty to a stretcher using a blanket

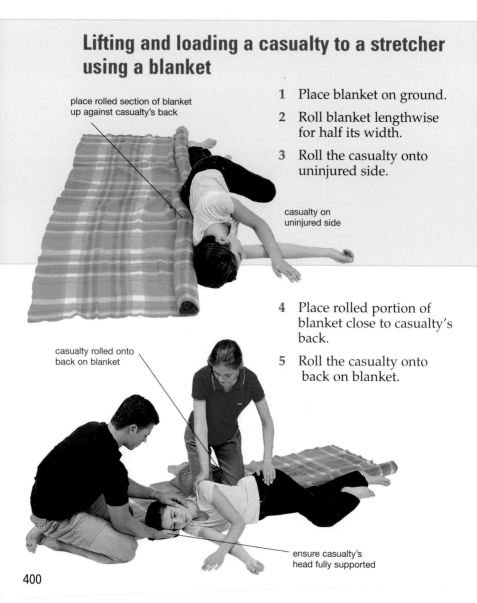

place rolled section of blanket up against casualty's back

casualty on uninjured side

casualty rolled onto back on blanket

ensure casualty's head fully supported

1 Place blanket on ground.

2 Roll blanket lengthwise for half its width.

3 Roll the casualty onto uninjured side.

4 Place rolled portion of blanket close to casualty's back.

5 Roll the casualty onto back on blanket.

6 Unroll the blanket.

7 To lift: roll up edges of blanket until alongside the casualty—edges act as handles for lifters. Grasp rolled edges firmly.

8 One lifter takes control, signalling when to lift.

9 All lifters rise at same time.

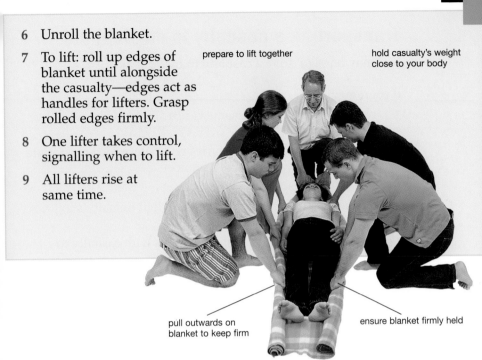

prepare to lift together

hold casualty's weight close to your body

pull outwards on blanket to keep firm

ensure blanket firmly held

Casualty lifted and placed on stretcher

Transporting a casualty to medical aid

You may have to drive a casualty to medical aid.

If so, remember:
- casualty still needs the same care as if they were not being moved
- the nature of casualty's injuries will determine appropriate vehicle to use (if you have a choice)
- not to exceed speed limit
- if necessary, travel slowly to ensure that casualty's injuries are not made worse
- the most experienced first aider stays with casualty to monitor airway.

Casualties suffering from the following conditions must always be transported on a stretcher:
- head injuries
- spinal injuries
- abdominal injuries
- lower limb injuries
- embedded foreign bodies or penetrating wounds to the eye.

Casualties with minor injuries and some upper limb injuries may be moved (preferably only short distances) sitting in a car, provided the injured parts are adequately supported.

First aid in the workplace

The responsibility of ensuring workplace safety rests with all employers and employees. All workplaces have hazards which may or may not be obvious. They may include aspects of the physical environment, materials and equipment used, and work practices.

Each State and Territory has a number of Acts, Regulations, Codes of Practice, Compliance Codes and Ordinances which regulate the work environment and provide minimum standards for the protection of workers' health and safety.

The role of the first aider in assisting with ongoing safety of workers and in managing injuries and illnesses is outlined in this chapter. Some legal responsibilities of employers, employees and the first aider are also discussed.

First aid in the workplace

First aider's responsibilities

The main role of the first aider in the workplace is to provide first aid management of illness and injury. Other responsibilities may include:

- record keeping
- recognition and reporting of health and safety hazards
- performing risk assessments
- participation in safety programs
- maintenance of a first aid kit and/or first aid room
- awareness of temporary and permanent staff injuries and illnesses.

Prevention of injury and illness should be of the utmost importance in every workplace. Injuries can cause much trauma and cost time and money. Unsafe working conditions lead to inefficiencies in production. Preventive first aid is a major part of the first aider's responsibilities.

Ongoing safety education is crucial for the prevention of accidents. Working according to safe practice guidelines, have proven to be efficient in the long term.

All workplaces have hazards. Chemicals, plant and machinery, tools and equipment, material handling and storage, electrical installations and radiation are obvious dangers. In workplaces such as offices, the dangers are not as obvious. Such conditions as stress or shock can present themselves in these low risk environments at any time, even if not caused directly by the work area.

Types of injury in the workplace

Back injuries comprise approximately one quarter of all injuries in the workplace and are the most frequently reported result of industrial accidents or manual handling practices. Such injuries cause physical suffering to the employee and cost employers millions of dollars in lost time and medical expenses.

Skin rashes, skin infections and allergic reactions to substances are also commonly reported in the workplace and comprise about 50% of occupational diseases. Various chemicals and other agents, and hot, humid work conditions are common causes
of rashes, allergic reactions and skin infections.

Contact dermatitis is one of the two main types of occupational skin rash. It may be caused by:

- physical irritants (e.g. friction, heat, moisture, ultraviolet light)
- chemical irritants (e.g. acids, alkalis, mercury compounds)
- fat solvents (e.g. thinners, formaldehyde).

Allergic dermatitis is the other main skin disease resulting from workplace conditions. It may result from sensitivities to oils and coal tars, rubber, dyes, resins and plastics and even soaps and cosmetics. Skin infections are caused by bacteria (e.g. staphylococcus aureus or 'golden staph' and fungi (e.g. tinea). Fungal infections are more common in hot, humid workplaces.

Radiation burns may be caused by the sun, welding arcs, ultraviolet rays or nuclear accidents, resulting in extensive superficial burns and blisters. Nuclear irradiation can also severely damage internal organs with consequences such as diarrhoea, vomiting and shock. Death may occur even after twenty-four hours.

Hearing damage can occur in workplaces where there is exposure to constant and/or a higher than normal levels of noise. Most States in Australia have legislation aimed at preserving the hearing of people working in such conditions and requiring the use of protective devices and monitoring employees' exposure.

Chest and blast injuries and amputation are likely to occur in particular types of workplaces. They usually result from accidents associated with heavy equipment and machinery.

Accidents with chemicals usually occur in the workplace when workers have a lack of awareness of safety precautions and do not use Personal Protective Equipment (PPE). First aiders should be familiar with chemicals used in the workplace and have access to up-to-date Material Safety Data Sheets (MSDS) for those chemicals. The MSDS provides information on the potential hazards and appropriate first aid management in the event of an emergency.

In the office environment, awareness of fire evacuation procedures and the location of the nearest fire extinguisher, first aid kit and first aider is essential.

Legal issues

State and Territory requirements

Legislation covering safety requirements in the workplace varies in States and Territories and in industries. Each State and Territory has an Occupational and Workplace Health and Safety Act and a number of other Acts, Ordinances and Regulations providing a set of minimum standards.

Legal issues arising from first aid in the workplace include:

- consent to treatment—a rational casualty can refuse first aid
- respect for casualty's privacy
- confidentiality of records
- destruction of records
- liability for improper or negligent administration of first aid.

Consent to first aid treatment

As a general rule, mentally competent adults have the right to refuse any treatment, even if that treatment is necessary to save their lives. Treatment given to a person without consent may constitute an assault.

Consent can be implied or expressed. If the casualty goes to the first aid room and cooperates with the first aid officer, consent is implied (taken as given). Consent is expressed when oral or written permission is given.

In some situations a person cannot give consent to treatment— for example, if the injury or illness has affected the ability to make an informed choice, if the casualty is unconscious, or is very young or mentally disabled. In these cases, consent is not required and a qualified person may administer any necessary treatment to save the person's life or to prevent serious illness or further injury.

Privacy and confidentiality

Legislation varies with respect to who can have access to first aid records, the extent of this access, and what incidents have to be reported. However, the following people have the right to access:

- ambulance officers or a treating doctor
- those investigating workplace illness or injury—police, coroner, workplace inspection authority, the courts
- employer (e.g. to ensure injury was work-related or to assist in identifying cause).

With the casualty's agreement, access is given to:

- the insurance company handling the claim
- union representatives or occupational health and safety committees.

Legislation also requires that occupational incidents causing serious injury or death be reported to the relevant government authority. Legislation may require the employer to report the incident, but the first aider is required to complete the notification.

Despite legitimate access by many people to first aid records, the privacy of the casualty should always be respected to the greatest extent possible. The person controlling the records has a responsibility to ensure they are only released to people with appropriate authority and all records must be stored in a secure location. The casualty should be informed if access has been given. A record should be kept of anyone who has had access to particular documents, and when and why.

Destruction of records

There are no national rules regarding destruction of records. However, your State or Territory Occupational Health and Safety legislation may specify a set of rules.

Liability

First aiders are only liable for any injury caused by them if
negligence can be shown. The person suing must be able to
show, among other things, a duty of care, and that the
treatment was not reasonable in the circumstances.

First aid rooms and kits

The relevant Acts/*Codes of Practice Guidelines* set out minimum
requirements for the availability and contents of first aid rooms
and kits. Extra equipment will vary according to hazards
associated with specific workplaces and industries. *States and
Territory Codes of Practice or Guidelines may also specify additional
items such as antiseptic, anti-itch or sunscreen preparations.*

First aid rooms

Laws, guidance from Codes of Practice or relevant Acts for the
specific requirements for first aid rooms and equipment are set
by each State and Territory. Minimum standards or guidelines
for first aid rooms can be obtained from your State or Territory
authorities and should be followed. Nominally a first aid room
would have:

- a minimum floor area of approximately 15 square metres
- good illumination and ventilation
- easy access to toilets
- access door wide enough to cater for a stretcher
  or wheelchair
- hot and cold running water
- adequate space for rendering first aid.

First aid kits

Generally, a first aid kit should be readily accessible to all those in the workplace. It should:

- be clearly marked with a white cross on a green background
- contain first aid instructions
- be dust and moisture proof
- be large enough to store all first aid requirements
- contain first aid instructions.

A first aid risk assessment should be conducted for the workplace. First aid kits and rooms must be stocked with supplies appropriate for managing injuries that may occur in the workplace, and all equipment must be maintained for operational readiness.

A notice giving the name and location of the person responsible for first aid should be placed on the kit or outside the first aid room. Depending on state/territory code of practice/guidelines, the first aider has the responsibility to ensure that:

- the first aid room is kept tidy and clean
- first aid stock is regularly checked and replenished
- medication is clearly labelled and stored as directed
- expiry dates are checked regularly.

Reporting illness and injury

The majority of Acts require deaths and various classes of accidents to be reported to the appropriate Government authority. First aiders should be aware of the documentation requirements of the Acts, Ordinances and Regulations relevant to their workplace.

Documentation

Employers are required to maintain a written record of all injuries and illnesses at the place of employment. Legislation may require that work-related injuries and illnesses are recorded on an accident report form *(see p. 413)* and in an accident register.

Accurate reporting and documentation of casualty information are important functions of the first aider. This applies to all incidents where workers seek advice or treatment relating to first aid. Maintenance of good, accurate records is necessary:

- for proper clinical management
- as the law requires such records
- to protect the first aider against possible litigation and prosecution
- to protect individuals if controversy ensues
- to protect the company
- to provide information for evaluation of injury and illness trends.

First aid record keeping

Documentation must be accurate and legible. It should include the employee's factual account of the incident, but not opinion and hearsay. Records should be written at the time treatment is given or as soon afterwards as possible. They must be written in ink or ballpoint and never erased. Mistakes must be crossed through and 'wrong entry' written next to them. Records of accidents should be validated and signed by the employee involved.

All medical records must be kept strictly confidential and should:

- be stored in a locked cupboard
- be accessible only to first aiders and authorised personnel
- not be made available to unauthorised personnel.

Types of records

The format of records varies between industries and between workplaces because of different policy requirements and legislation.

Referral letters

Where employees are referred to a doctor or hospital, referral letters should accompany them giving:

- brief personal details (name, date of birth, address, job, allergies, previous medical history)
- date of referral
- history of injury/illness (what happened, when and where)
- observations (what seen/felt) and vital signs
- first aider's assessment of injury/illness
- first aid management (wound dressings, medication, referral)
- signature and status of first aider.

If a chemical or toxic substance has been involved, all information should accompany the casualty to the doctor or hospital.

Injury report

An injury report is a full account of what happened as related by the casualty. It should have sufficient information to satisfy statutory requirements. A copy of this report is given to the supervisor and safety officer.

EMPLOYER

Name
_____

Industry
_____

Phone
_____

Address
_____

_____

_____

WORK INJURY
REPORT FORM

INJURED PERSON

Full Name: _____ Age: _____ Sex: _____

Residential Address: _____

Trade or Occupation: _____

Industry in which the person was working at the time of injury:
_____

Activity in which the person was engaged at the time of injury:
_____

Date and time injury occurred:

Date: _____ Day: _____ Time: _____ AM/PM

INJURY – Brief description of the type and cause of the injury, the part of the body injured and the treatment given.

_____

_____

_____

_____

Name of the person rendering first aid: (Please print)

Name: _____ Signature: _____

Details of any referral or further treatment:

_____

_____

_____

PERSON COMPLETING REPORT

Name: _____ Phone Number: _____

_____ Date: _____
(Block letters)

Signature: _____

Note: 1. Company should ensure that sufficient information is included to satisfy statutory requirements.
2. It may be appropriate to include company's privacy statement.

FIRST AID IN THE WORKPLACE

20

Daily attendance register

A first aider should also maintain a daily attendance register. This contains a summary of all casualties seen during each shift, each entry being signed by the first aider. This register may be perused in court, sometimes years after an initial injury or illness.

Injury statistics

Injury statistics are a summary of illnesses and injuries occurring in a workplace over a given time. Statistics are useful in detecting trends and can be used to prevent accidents, reduce their severity, and evaluate safety procedures.

More detailed information on first aid in the workplace can be found in the *St John Ambulance Occupational First Aid* publication.

21

Emotionally disturbed casualties

First aiders sometimes need to care for casualties who are in severe emotional distress. The distress may be due to a range of factors, or a combination of the casualty's baseline mental health or emotional state; the effect of drugs or alcohol; and the natural physical and psychological reactions following an accident.

Most casualties are frightened; and many are in pain. This modifies their interaction with others and those who are there to help. Some casualties have a basic psychiatric illness which in itself is the cause of their needing first aid or medical help.

Aggressive, angry or violent behaviour may also be a consequence of deeply distressing and fearful emotions. The first aider needs to be able to respond appropriately when confronted by people experiencing extreme distress. First aiders need to be able to cope with this situation while, at the same time, assisting the casualty and possibly others at the scene until professional help arrives. Communication skills, especially listening, and observation are your greatest assets. The first aider and casualty's body language are important. Imparting confidence and controlling the incident or accident site is very important. This chapter discusses the more common types of severe emotional distress and the first aider's role in their management.

Psychological trauma

Every person who has faced a threat to life or limb shows signs of fear. Psychological reactions usually accompany physical injury, particularly when the injury is the result of serious accidents, criminal assault, natural disasters, war or community violence.

Children are keen observers and realise that something is wrong even if no one talks to them about it. If they are not given the facts, they will fill in the blanks with their imagination. They sometimes assume that a crisis or tragedy was their fault and in some cases the child's fantasies may be scarier than what actually happened. Young and older children often react to trauma in physical ways. A young child thinks and feels but doesn't have the skills to articulate their thoughts and feelings to their parents or carers. Sometimes stress reactions surface weeks or even months after a traumatic event. Every child reacts differently and may not react the way that an adult expects.

Acute stress reaction

Traumatic events involving intense fear, horror, helplessness or violation often produce an acute stress reaction—a syndrome which may comprise palpations, over-breathing or a wide range of signs (see below). Acute stress reactions vary from individual to individual. Different individuals have different 'threshold points'. Casualties are more likely to recover from an acute stress reaction if the first aider is confident, calm, competent and compassionate. The first aider will greatly help by providing practical assistance and by caring, listening and giving information.

SIGNS AND SYMPTOMS

The signs and symptoms of acute stress reaction are caused by the flooding of the mind with continuous and uncontrollable thoughts that result in emotional, cognitive and physical responses. Children may manifest physical reactions and these depend on a wide range of factors including their age, their stage of development and the way in which the adults around them are handling the event.

Signs and symptoms of acute stress include:
- shock, disbelief, numbness, fear, feeling as though what happened is unreal
- shortness of breath, dizziness, hyperventilation
- palpitations, chest pain
- hot and cold flushes, sweating
- tension, uncontrollable tremor
- nausea and vomiting, diarrhoea
- confusion, inability to concentrate.

Management of acute stress reaction

1 If the casualty's physical state permits, remove them to a quiet, safe spot, preferably out of sight of fearful or upsetting scenes.

2 Reassure the casualty of his or her safety and encourage rest.

3 Help the casualty to make contact with family members or friends. This may include telephone calls or being positioned near people that they know.

4 Be a good listener—if appropriate, allow the casualty to talk about what happened and how they are feeling to provide relief. It is alright to remain silent and to reassure by acknowledging the distress of the current situation.

5 Try to anticipate needs (e.g. drink, warmth, food, family). Perhaps ask specifically if they need a drink or need to contact someone.

DO NOT interrupt, reassure falsely, try to talk casualty out of these feelings, recount your own experiences or say that others are worse off.

6 Stay calm, connected and understanding to the limit that you are able.

DO NOT take it personally if the casualty is angry or blames others.

7 After the casualty has talked about what happened, reassure that their feelings and the way that they are thinking is normal after such as incident.

8 If the casualty cannot talk about what happened or express feelings, sit quietly and give support by your presence.

Post-traumatic stress disorder

Post-traumatic stress disorder (PTSD) is a serious psychological reaction that develops in some people following exposure to an overwhelming, frightening or traumatic event.

In some cases, the symptoms of stress can persist for several weeks and the symptoms can begin to interfere with the person's normal life activities such as working, relationships and recreation. The persistence of these symptoms may be medically diagnosed as post-traumatic stress. Such casualties may require ongoing medical and professional treatment. It is important that the first aider only provide emotional first aid to ease or reduce the symptoms and does not make any comments about the diagnosis or use such psychiatric terms as 'post-traumatic stress'.

The symptoms of PTSD can be intrusive (intense recurring memories or dreams), avoidance (withdrawing from people or situations to stop the traumatic memories) or excessive arousal with a person constantly on guard and wary of potential dangers. Often special sounds (bangs, cries) or smells (e.g. cooking meat) may trigger instant 'flash backs'. They might experience problems with sleeping and concentration.

By offering calm, compassionate support and first aid treatment at the time of the incident, the first aider can help to minimise both acute stress reactions and the risk of PTSD developing later.

Grief

Grief is a normal response to loss. This might be a physical loss or a loss of lifestyle or essential activity. People grieve in different ways and there is no right or wrong way to grieve. People's responses to loss depend on individual factors such as personality, age, and relationship with the deceased; and on local or family or cultural practices including the level of personal or social support. Spiritual beliefs are very important. There are various stages within the grieving process which include denial, anger, despair, and the questioning of values and beliefs; before final acceptance. Grief includes a wide range of emotions, thoughts and behaviours but it doesn't help to think that grief will happen in a particular order which everyone moves through in a predictable way.

The range of normal reactions include:
- shock and disbelief
- loneliness, despair
- helplessness
- guilt and remorse
- feeling unable to cope
- confusion, anger or denial
- relief.

Management of grief

Expressions of grief, being emotional and personal and individual, can be difficult for the first aider to manage. It is important that first aiders recognise their capacity to assist in this situation. If a first aider is in a position to assist a person who is expressing grief, the following actions may be useful:

1   Provide a quiet supportive place for the person to be able to express their emotions (e.g. crying, coming to terms with an initial shock).

2   If possible reconnect the person with people (family members, friends) known to them.

3   If appropriate, encourage the person to express their thoughts and feelings by being a willing listener.

Psychiatric casualties

Always treat people with a psychiatric illness (or those who are impaired by drugs or alcohol) with the same politeness and respect, and compassionate firmness with which you treat others. Although casualties may appear thought-disordered or violent, they usually remember the details of the situation—sometimes with extreme embarrassment or shame—and the treatment given. Wherever possible reassure accompanying family, friends and onlookers, who also may be confused or deeply upset.

General management

Protect yourself and others from getting hurt. Do not get closely involved unless you are convinced it is safe.

1   If you judge it is not safe, **call 000** for emergency services.

    If you judge it is safe:

    • approach the casualty and identify yourself as a first aider.

2   Check vital signs, if casualty gives you permission to do so.

3   Check the casualty's level of consciousness by asking name, address, date, and whereabouts.

4   Stay calm, positive and open. Be polite and respectful.

5   Encourage the casualty to tell you what is on their mind. Listen closely.

6   Do not interrupt, contradict, argue, or falsely reassure casualty. Don't scold, slap, or attempt to restrain the casualty.

7   **Call 000** for emergency services when you have enough information.

Panic

SIGNS AND SYMPTOMS

- anxiety, fear, terror
- rapid breathing, breathlessness, sometimes hyperventilation to the point of spasms
- racing heart, cold sweaty palms, enlarged pupils, tremor
- headache, lump in the throat, a feeling of constriction or pain in the chest
- diarrhoea
- frequency of urination.

Management of panic

1 Move the casualty to a quiet place.

2 Calm the casualty by attentive listening, helping them relax, and encouraging them to slow breathing in unison with your own.

3 Stay with the casualty until medical aid arrives.

Depression and suicidal behaviour

SIGNS AND SYMPTOMS

- sadness, dejection, self-blame, despair, hopelessness
- suicidal ideas; e.g. hinting or even saying explicitly that they will kill themselves
- slow movements, decreased or increased appetite, weight loss or gain, insomnia, loss of interest in activities
- sudden dramatic change such as from sadness and hopelessness to apparent resolution and happiness may be a sign of impending suicide
- a real suicide attempt—however ineffectual this may seem (e.g. tablets, cutting).

Management of depression and suicidal behaviour

1 Always take any threats of suicide seriously.

2 If the situation is life-threatening or dangerous, ask someone to **call 000**.

3 Identify yourself as a first aider.

4 Check vital signs, if the casualty gives you consent.

5 Check level of consciousness—ask name, address, date and whereabouts.

6 Encourage the casualty to talk—listen and remain open, be polite and respectful.

7 Attempt to ascertain whether casualty has suicidal ideas or has taken an overdose.

8 Stay with casualty until help arrives.

Thought disorder

Thought disorders occur in such conditions as schizophrenia, bipolar disorder (manic-depressive psychosis) or those casualties affected by drugs. Most people with severe mental illness are not violent. They are more likely to be confused, wandering, out-of-touch, or withdrawn.

SIGNS AND SYMPTOMS

- disorganised thinking, racing thoughts, emotions not consistent with reality
- hearing or seeing things that are not there (i.e. hallucinations and delusions)
- odd or false ideas (e.g. that some group or person is following them).

Management of thought disorder

1. **Call 000** for emergency services.

2. Approach casualty quietly—identify yourself as a first aider.

3. Be polite and respectful. Stay calm, yet firm and in control.

4. Assure the casualty that help is on the way.

5. Ask for consent to monitor vital signs.

6. Check state of consciousness—ask name, address, date and whereabouts.

7. Allow the casualty to talk—listen attentively.

8. Do not interrupt, contradict or debate the casualty's ideas, however bizarre they may seem.

9. Stay with casualty until help arrives.

Violence

Violent behaviour can result from any one or a combination of factors. These include intoxication from alcohol or drugs, mental illness in which the casualty fears attack and acts in self-defence, domestic disputes and physical illness (e.g. low blood sugar).

SIGNS AND SYMPTOMS

- defensive, excited, threatening, belligerent, argumentative
- may have a weapon
- may be or appear to be intoxicated
- shouting or talking to unseen images.

Management of violence

1 **Call 000** for emergency services.

2 DO NOT put yourself in danger.

   Protect others from getting hurt.

   DO NOT approach the casualty unless you judge it is safe.

   DO NOT approach a casualty who has a weapon.

   NEVER try to force a weapon from a casualty.

3 If you decide it is safe, approach casualty slowly from the front. Avoid staring at or towering over the casualty. Sit down with them if you think it is safe.

4 Speak gently and identify yourself as a first aider. Allow the casualty to talk. Be polite and respectful.

5 Check vital signs if casualty gives you consent.

6 Check casualty's state of consciousness—ask name, address, date and whereabouts.

7 Try to ascertain source of casualty's anger. Fear, grief, humiliation, rejection or depression may be at the root of the problem.

8 Stay with casualty until help arrives.

21

22

Drug and alcohol misuse

Drug and alcohol misuse, either accidental or deliberate, may lead to intoxication or poisoning. The personal and social costs of substance abuse are enormous and include disability, and loss of good health and even life. These result in increased health care costs, and loss of productivity.

Legal and illegal substances are implicated in a significant number of hospital admissions, child abuse cases, suicides, road accident deaths, assaults, domestic violence, family disruption and crime.

Illnesses range from ruptured stomach linings and peptic ulcers to heart disease, liver disease and brain damage. Injuries result from vehicle crashes, pedestrian rundowns, drowning, interpersonal violence and sexual assault.

This chapter discusses the management of casualties suffering effects of substance use and misuse, the signs and symptoms of their misuse and some aspects of the associated health costs.

Substance use, dependence and addiction

The term 'drug' describes substances which, when taken, cause some specific or abnormal physical or mental change. Drugs may be swallowed, injected or inhaled for many reasons including pain relief, to promote recovery from illness, for other medicinal purposes, for pleasure, for peer group approval, and to escape from problems. Drugs include legal substances such as alcohol, tobacco, and prescribed and over-the-counter medication, as well as those which are illegal.

Whether the substance is legal or illegal, the use of some drugs can lead to dependency and addiction. In the case of alcohol, drugs of addiction and some stimulants, the more often they are taken, the less effective they are on the body because the body builds up a tolerance to them or gets rid of them quicker. The result may be that casualties or users keep increasing the dose to achieve the same effect.

A person is dependent on a substance when the substance is needed to function normally (e.g. insulin for a diabetic), or when the person feels it is needed.

Dependency on drugs may be purely psychological (e.g. a craving for tobacco or coffee) which is referred to as habituation. If to this psychological craving is added the element of physical dependency, then one speaks of a true addiction. In this latter case, the addict needs to absorb the drug continuously and in increasing doses to prevent the appearance or development of uncontrollable physical signs. The sudden stopping of drugs or alcohol to someone who is either habituated or addicted is referred to as 'going cold turkey'.

Those with a dependence on a substance, who develop an overwhelming and uncontrollable physical or psychological craving for it, have an addiction.

When a person with an addiction to a substance, stops using it, withdrawal symptoms will occur. This causes severe mental and physical distress, including such symptoms as irritability, aggression, anger and restlessness. Withdrawal from some drugs of addiction, including alcohol, produces delerium tremens or the 'DTs' which may be associated with seizures and death.

Effects of substance use and misuse

Substance misuse may be:

- accidental (e.g. taking too much of a substance or the wrong dose)
- deliberate (e.g. for social or emotional reasons or with suicidal intent).

Accidental substance use and misuse

A person may accidentally misuse a substance when:

- too much is taken (overdose)
- too little is taken
- taking of a dose is forgotten so another is taken
- two substances are taken which interact to produce unintended harmful effects.

The effects of accidental misuse range from not very serious to life-threatening. Misuse of drugs and their consequences differ from the risk of side effects (e.g. diarrhoea, nausea or rash) or unintended effects from a substance. Such side effects may result from a sensitivity to the substance.

People most at risk of accidental substance misuse are:

- those who regularly take a number of medications
- those who take other people's medication
- those who experiment with substances
- children (due to curiosity or normal toddler experimentation or mistaking medication for lollies or drinks)
- the elderly.

People may take multiple doses of their medication if they become confused. This is more likely to happen if:

- the person is taking a number of substances
- containers or medication are changed
- directions are not detailed or clear
- the person is not aware what condition the medication is for.

Deliberate substance use and misuse

In Australia, the most used and misused substances are alcohol and tobacco. Although the initial effects of these 'social' drugs are usually pleasurable, there are dangers associated with their use. Pharmaceuticals may also be misused when people take a cocktail of medications with alcohol, or overuse analgesic medications.

The commonest method of suicide is to ingest drugs or poisons. The amount taken may be just enough to gain attention—a 'cry for help'—or enough to cause death.

Effects

The immediate effects of substance misuse are usually nausea, vomiting and acute diarrhoea. Failing respiration, irregular heartbeat and unconsciousness may follow. Longer-term effects may be damage to the kidneys, liver, lungs and brain.

The wider impact of substance misuse includes social effects such as accidents (e.g. drowning, car accidents), aggression, family disruption, absenteeism, disdain by colleagues and crime to maintain a drug habit.

Risk management

Occasionally, casualties who are under the influence of alcohol or drugs may be at risk of harming themselves or others through dangerous or violent behaviour.

In handling such a situation:

DO NOT put yourself at risk.

DO NOT approach the casualty if you do not feel it is safe.

DO NOT be judgmental (you could provoke hostility).

Management of substance misuse

1 Follow **DRABCD**.

- **Danger**—risk management

- **Response**—what is level of consciousness?

- **Airway**—be mindful of risk to airway from vomiting

- **Breathing**—consider oxygen therapy with resuscitation equipment if necessary

- **CPR**—if no signs of life, give CPR

- **Defibrillation**—if no signs of life are present apply a defibrillator (if available).

2 **Call 000** for an ambulance.

3 Be calm, reassuring and act professionally; quietly move the casualty to safety if necessary.

4 Be aware of the possibility of infectious diseases (e.g. contaminated needles)—follow 'standard precautions' to avoid infection *(see p. 133)*.

5 Remove any potential missiles and weapons from the vicinity if possible.

6 Seek information:

- history—gain information about what, when, and how much the casualty has taken or used

- observations—monitor vital signs frequently (including conscious state).

7 Check for possible fractures or other injuries—give appropriate first aid.

8 Attempt to keep vomit, or at least a sample, to send with casualty to hospital.

9 Keep substances or containers for identification—send with casualty to hospital.

Commonly misused substances

Stimulants

Stimulants increase a person's feelings of excitement and promote energy, at least in the short term. In some, they may produce a transient feeling of happiness and increased confidence. In others, they may cause anxiety. Stimulants affect the nervous system, speeding up mental and physical activity, making the person feel more alert and more able to perform a task.

Depending on the type of stimulant, use may produce over-stimulation, exhilaration, excitability, visual disturbances, hallucinations and delusions. This is usually followed by a period of depression or 'let down'.

SIGNS AND SYMPTOMS

Signs of the use of stimulants may include an increase in pulse, increased respiration and raised temperature, sweating, irritability, nausea, vomiting and odd behaviour.

Stimulants may be swallowed, sniffed, injected or inhaled. They include:

- amphetamines (also called 'speed', 'ice')
- cocaine (also referred to as 'coke')
- ecstasy (also referred to as 'E').

Legal substances which act as stimulants, especially when overused, include:

- caffeine products such as coffee, tea, and some soft drinks
- nicotine
- prescription drugs for weight loss and behaviour disorders.

Hallucinogens

Hallucinogens alter perception of ordinary stimuli and cause changes in mood, emotions, sensation and self-awareness. They can alter the person's perceptions of time and space, and produce delusions. During a 'bad trip', the person may feel intense fear, panic, profound depression, tension and anxiety.

The most common hallucinogens are:
- lysergic acid diethylamide (LSD or 'acid')
- certain types of mushrooms (e.g. gold tops)
- phencyclidine (PCP, 'angel dust')
- mescaline (peyote or buttons)
- marijuana, hashish.

Depressants

Depressants affect the central nervous system, slowing down mental and physical activity. They are usually swallowed as tablets, liquids or powder but may occasionally be inhaled or injected. Depressant drugs usually affect the 'higher' centres of the brain first. This may result in disinhibition inhibition when a person's normal sensitivities and self control are depressed, thus temporarily allowing the more instinctual or 'baser' drives or instincts to surface. Alcohol is the best example of this.

The principal dangers of depressants are impairment of coordination and judgment, and ultimately, depression of all body functions including consciousness, heart function, blood pressure and respiration. Oxygen therapy may be of particular need in first aid treatment when depressants have been misused.

Common depressants include:

- alcohol
- barbiturates (or other sleeping tablets)
- benzodiazepines (or other tranquillisers)
- narcotics (e.g. heroin, methadone or pethidine)
- volatile inhalants (e.g. petrol, thinners, glue).

Pharmaceuticals

Casualties who have accidentally or deliberately overdosed on pharmaceuticals have often taken a combination of drugs that affect their level of consciousness.

It is important to summon help quickly. If he or she can do so with safety, the first aider should try to prevent the casualty taking any more drugs, and to be ready to resuscitate, if necessary, until help arrives.

Paracetamol

Paracetamol is a general purpose painkiller for mild to moderate pain. Special care is needed for its use in children. There is a narrow 'window' between its effective dose and its toxic dose. Too much paracetamol can cause serious, potentially fatal, liver damage. DO NOT deviate from the prescribed dosage. Always read the directions on the packaging before administering this medication.

Children and drugs or medications

Accidental poisoning

The most common cause of poisoning in young children is swallowing medication or household products which have not been stored safely.

Management of substance poisoning—child

1 DO NOT make the child vomit—this can cause further harm.

2 If the child does vomit, keep vomitus to show the doctor.

3 DO NOT give fluids—this will dilute the substance and may hasten absorption.

4 Call the Poisons Information Centre—13 11 26.

5 Reassure the child.

6 Gently ask the child:

- how much substance was swallowed

- when substance were taken.

7 Seek medical aid according to the advice from the Poisons Information Centre.

If the child is becoming drowsy or is unconscious:

1 **Call 000** for an ambulance.

2 Open the child's mouth and hook out with a finger any substance you can see.

3 Place the child on his or her side in the recovery position and monitor airway and breathing regularly.

Alcohol

SIGNS AND SYMPTOMS

Even a small amount of alcohol can be harmful to a young child. Signs and symptoms that a child has drunk alcohol are:

- strong smell of alcohol
- flushed moist face
- slurred speech
- staggering
- deep noisy breathing
- nausea
- pounding pulse.

Management of alcohol ingestion—child

1 Seek medical aid if the child is drunk, is becoming drowsy or is unconscious.

2 Allow child to rest; help lie in recovery position.

3 Examine the bottle or ask the child how much he or she has drunk.

4 Place a bowl near the child in case of vomiting.

5 If the child goes to sleep, check regularly that the child can be roused easily.

6 If the child is unconscious, place him or her on their side in the recovery position and monitor airway and breathing regularly.

23

Childbirth

Most expectant parents will have attended classes to prepare themselves for the birth of their baby. Nevertheless, all parents expecting their first child or mothers-to-be who have gone into labour unexpectedly need special support.

Remaining calm and reassuring the expectant mother will help her to stay calm. This will help her to remember the procedures she has been taught and to deal with the labour more comfortably.

Labour usually lasts for several hours and in most cases proceeds normally. There is generally plenty of time to arrange for transport to hospital or to seek medical assistance.

This chapter outlines the procedures for delivering a baby safely, even when the birth is not entirely straightforward.

Childbirth preparation

Childbirth is a natural process and the majority of babies are born without complications during delivery. First aid assistance may be necessary if the baby starts to come before its due time, if the woman lives in a remote part of the country or if an emergency occurs which threatens the life of the mother or the baby. In any of these situations, assistance with the delivery of the baby and care for the mother may be necessary until an ambulance, midwife or medical practitioner arrives.

Note: If you encounter a birth away from medical assistance or access to an ambulance service, call for urgent medical advice, using a telephone, mobile phone, or Royal Flying Doctor Service radio for continuing advice during delivery.

Infection

Infection is a serious danger to both mother and baby.
It is essential to minimise the risk of infection:

- wash your hands, nails and forearms thoroughly with warm water and soap (if possible)
- wear disposable gloves if available.

Preparing for the birth

Childbirth is a very personal and emotional time for the parents, and may also be for the first aider. Preparation is essential, as well as calmness and reassurance.

The expectant mother will experience pain and strong emotions, and will have to work hard to deliver the baby. She may feel afraid, not know what to expect and want the support of someone close to her (such as the baby's father or a female friend). There will be blood and probably noise during the birth and she will need assistance to maintain her breathing pattern to aid the birth.

For the birth, the expectant mother can safely be delivered on any flat surface, although if she finds this uncomfortable, she may wish to squat or adopt some other comfortable position. If in a public area, ask others to move away to give the mother privacy. As a first aider, you can:

1 Prepare a suitable clean surface for the mother:
   - large plastic sheet to go under her
   - clean sheet to place over the plastic.
2 Boil water to sterilise the scissors for cutting the cord.
3 Collect other materials needed.

The first aider's childbirth kit

The following items are desirable in preparation for the birth but unlikely to be available in an emergency—do the best you can:

- 1 large plastic sheet
- 2 clean cotton sheets
- 3 bunny rugs
- towels
- large plastic bags for soiled linen
- 3 sterile or clean cord ties (e.g. string, linen tape) each about 8 cm long
- sterile scissors
- gauze swabs or a clean soft cloth
- sanitary pads/disposable nappies
- disposable gloves
- large plastic bag for placenta.

The birth

First stage—onset of labour

The first stage of labour usually lasts less than 12 hours. However, a woman who has already had a child may progress through this stage very rapidly—sometimes, seemingly in less than 30 minutes. Early contractions may begin as an aching feeling in the lower abdomen.

Signs—first stage

Signs usually include one or all of the following:

- cramp-like pains in lower abdomen every 2–15 minutes, each lasting 30–60 seconds increasing in frequency and duration
- a 'show' of bloodstained mucus—the plug which sealed the cervix during pregnancy—may occur up to a few days before the onset of labour

- the 'waters breaking'—a sudden rush, or sometimes a constant trickle, of amniotic fluid indicates the sac containing the baby has broken; note the colour and consistency and inform medical aid.

Management of first stage

1 Reassure the pregnant mother.

2 Keep her comfortable.

3 **Call 000** for an ambulance.

4 If the ambulance will be delayed, begin to collect the materials needed.

Note: Many expectant mothers in early labour become very restless. As this first stage may take a number of hours, she may wish to move around.

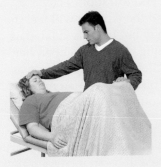

Preparation for second stage

1 Assist the expectant mother into a comfortable position. If the woman is most comfortable on her back, then ensure her upper body is raised.

2 Help in removing any clothing that may be in the way during delivery. Warm baby blankets (bunny rugs).

Second stage—the birth

The second stage begins when the cervix (neck of the womb) is fully dilated (widened) and ends with the birth of the baby.

There are a number of potential dangers for the mother and baby during the birth.

Mother:

- bleeding
- infection.

Baby:

- lack of oxygen
- cold
- infection from the cut end of umbilical cord.

Signs—second stage

Contractions may alter in frequency and duration. They become quite intense at this stage and the woman will feel the urge to 'bear down'. As the cervix may not be fully dilated at this stage, discourage her from pushing. Ask her to open her mouth and pant during each contraction until help arrives as the baby is usually safer inside than out. The woman may push anyway either voluntary or involuntary.

Most babies are born head first. As the baby is about to be born, the top of the head can be seen at the opening to the birth canal. This is called 'crowning'. There will be an increased flow of bloodstained mucus and the mother may feel the need to have a bowel movement. DO NOT let her sit on the toilet.

Management of second stage

First aider's preparations

1 Tie an apron or sheet around first aider's waist to protect clothing and minimise infection.

2 Wash and dry hands thoroughly and put on disposable gloves if available.

3 Prepare two warmed blankets, towels or nappies for the baby.

Prepare expectant mother for delivery

1 Wash the area from the entrance to the vagina to the anus using soap and water and a clean swab for each stroke (wipe from front to back).

2 When head is crowning, encourage the mother to:

- stop pushing

- keep her mouth open and pant (fast, shallow breaths), as the baby's head is delivering

- rest between contractions.

Normal delivery with head presenting first

1 Control baby's head with gentle but steady pressure from the direction of the mother's pubic area downwards—the head will usually appear with the face towards the mother's anus but will then rotate to face one side.

2 Check whether umbilical cord is around the baby's neck:

- if cord is around the neck, free it by easing it carefully over the baby's head if at all possible (but do not pull on it)

- if this is not possible, try to slip the cord over the shoulder and deliver the baby through the cord. If it is not possible to do this, because the cord is too tight (a very rare event), it will be necessary to tie the cord in two places very firmly using sterile string or similar and then cut between the two ties (use sterile scissors).

3 Support the baby's head in palms of your hands and wait.

4 Once you can see the top shoulder, guide the head downwards to clear the shoulder from under the pubic bone. During the next contraction, both the baby's shoulders will be delivered. When the shoulders are out:

- encircle baby's chest with your hands to guide the baby out—do not pull

- lift baby up towards mother's stomach.

5 Note the time baby was born.

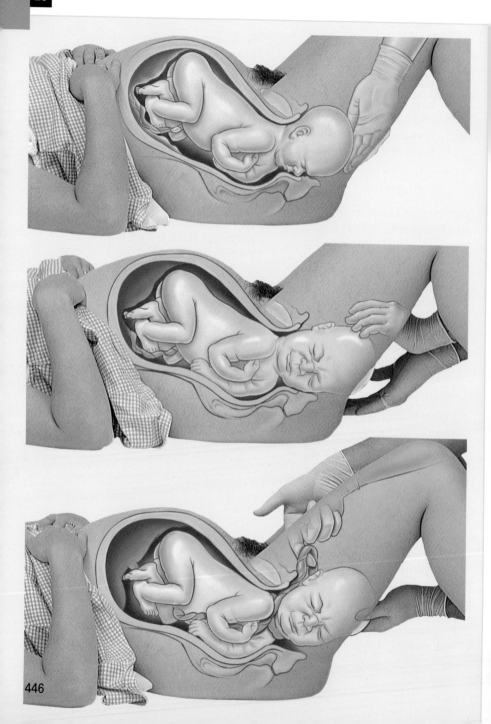

Management of second stage—complications

Delivery with buttocks or foot presenting first (breech birth)

This can become life-threatening for the baby if the head gets stuck in the birth canal after the body has been delivered. The umbilical cord will be compressed between the head and the walls of the vagina, and the baby will die from lack of oxygen.

1 Place mother in a position (for example on the very edge of bed) that allows the baby to be delivered downwards. **DO NOT PULL THE BABY**.

2 Allow mother to push the baby out herself—gently guide baby to ensure the back remains uppermost.

3 After delivery of hips and legs, wrap body of baby in a warm blanket.

4 After delivery of shoulders allow the baby to 'hang' downwards whilst being supported.

5 When the nape of the neck is visible:

- lift the baby's body upwards by the ankles, while supporting the body

- allow the head to deliver slowly.

Delivery with umbilical cord presenting first

This is a life-threatening situation because the cord will be compressed and the flow of oxygenated blood to the baby stopped. The baby could die within minutes.

1 Place mother in a kneeling position with head down and buttocks right up in the air.

2 Seek urgent medical advice.

3 Try to push the head up off the cord and gently replace the cord in the vagina. Handle the cord as little as possible as it may spasm.

Note: Inform mother of seriousness of this situation.

Immediate care of the baby

Immediately after birth, the baby will be wet and slippery. Take care not to drop the baby or pull on the cord. The baby may be blue at birth and must be kept warm. Leave the umbilical cord intact and, supporting the baby's head, neck and shoulders with one hand, and feet with the other:

- place baby's head low to drain secretions from mouth and nose

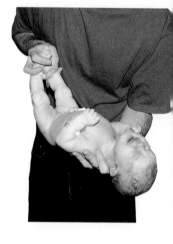

- dry baby quickly and thoroughly with a warm, clean towel

- if no resuscitation is necessary—place baby on mother's stomach skin to skin with a warm wrap over baby and encourage baby to breast-feed, this aids with keeping baby warm and provides maternal bonding

- wrap baby in warmed towel or blanket to keep it warm.

Most babies will cry straightaway, an indication of breathing. As they start breathing, they change from blue to pink (the hands and feet may remain blue for several hours).

If the baby does not breathe straightaway, try stimulating it by gently rubbing its back. DO NOT hold the baby upside down by the heels and slap it on the back or the buttocks to make it cry.

If the baby does not cry or show signs of breathing after 1 minute, clear the airway of mucus with your little finger and perform rescue breaths. To perform rescue breaths on a baby, seal your mouth over the mouth and nose together. Blow gently, just enough to see the chest rise— 30 breaths per minute.

In such cases inflation is nearly always the primary need of the newborn, not chest compression. Chest compressions on a newborn should NOT be attempted by persons untrained in neonatal resuscitation. The pulse is difficult to measure in the newborn but may be detectable by lightly holding the base of the umbilical cord between the thumb and index finger.

Third stage—the afterbirth

The afterbirth (placenta) is normally not delivered until 10 minutes or more after the birth of the baby. It is expelled by contractions of the uterus.

Management of the third stage—the afterbirth

To help delivery of afterbirth:

1   Help mother into a comfortable position, as for the birth.

2   If cord is long enough, encourage mother to put baby to her breast (this will help uterus to contract, expelling afterbirth and controlling bleeding)—DO NOT PULL ON CORD as this may cause excessive bleeding.

3   Retain afterbirth in a plastic bag for medical inspection.

4   Give mother hot or cold drinks and offer a light snack (provided afterbirth has been delivered).

After delivery of the afterbirth, the mother will bleed enough to fill a normal sanitary pad every 10–15 minutes for the first hour or so.

If there is a great deal of blood or the flow is not slowing down or it increases suddenly:

* **call 000** for an ambulance (if not already summoned)

* massage the top of the uterus until it becomes firm. It is usually located as high as the level of the umbilicus even after delivery—this will help reduce excessive bleeding.

Care of the mother

Once the mother has given birth, she will feel exhausted and may have 'the shakes'. Depending on circumstances and her wishes, the following will help her regain strength and minimise risk of infection:

- clean birth canal area with clean towels or gauze pads—wash the pubic area from front to back
- sponge her face, hands and legs and help her to change any soiled clothing
- place a sanitary pad or disposable nappy in position
- give her hot or cold drinks and offer a light snack (provided afterbirth has been delivered)
- cover her with a warm blanket
- check her pulse, temperature and respiration
- check blood loss regularly—gently massage lower abdomen to control excessive bleeding
- encourage her to rest while waiting for medical aid.

Once mother and baby have been cared for:

- retain all bloodstained material in plastic bags for medical inspection—separate bags for used sanitary pads
- clean all surfaces contaminated by blood and body fluids.

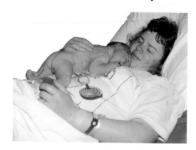

Care of the umbilical cord

Once the baby is pink and breathing, it does not need the blood supply from umbilical cord. After delivery of afterbirth, tie the cord only if there is a long delay expected before the arrival of the ambulance.

If the cord has to be tied:

1   Firmly tie with sterile string (e.g. bootlaces) in 3 places—10 cm, 15 cm and 20 cm from the baby's navel—cord must be tied securely to prevent bleeding after it is cut. As cutting the cord increases risk of bleeding and infection, it is necessary only if:

- there are complications during delivery *(see p. 447)*
- baby needs to be resuscitated and must be moved away from the mother
- mother needs attention and cannot hold baby
- cord is too short for mother to hold baby properly
- birth is in a remote area which is isolated from medical aid.

If the cord has to be cut:

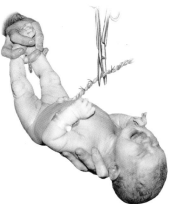

1   Cut between the 2nd and 3rd tie away from the baby.

2   Cover stump of the cord loosely with a sterile dressing.

3   Check cord for bleeding every 15 minutes for first hour then half hourly until medical aid arrives.

Vaginal bleeding and miscarriage

Miscarriage is the loss of the foetus before the twentieth week of pregnancy. This usually occurs because the foetus was not developing properly and was not able to survive.

A woman who miscarries is in danger of going into shock. She may be frightened and very distressed and reluctant to accept the help of a male first aider.

SIGN AND SYMPTOMS

- vaginal bleeding—this may be severe
- signs of shock
- cramp-like pains in lower abdomen
- aching in lower back
- expelling of foetus or tissue.

Management of miscarriage

1 **Call 000** for an ambulance.

2 Help her into a comfortable position.

3 Have her place towel or sanitary pad over her vulva.

4 Monitor bleeding (do not try to control) and pulse— record details every 10 minutes.

5 Help to maintain normal body temperature.

6 Keep any expelled material and give to medical personnel.

7 Do not give anything to eat or drink as she may need an operation.

24

Triage

Triage

Triage is defined as the process of sorting casualties and setting priorities for treatment. The aim is to establish priority for care of each casualty, to assist in the allocation of resources and the management and evacuation of the scene. A fundamental goal is for the greatest good to be done for the greatest number of people.

Triage areas should be distinctly marked and the site control centre well protected. It should be positioned so as to provide good access both to casualties and evacuation routes.

Multi-casualty road traffic accident

A major traffic accident may involve multiple casualties. At any accident site, first aid management will be limited by the resources available. This is particularly the case when there are a large number of casualties. In rural areas, people involved in a traffic accident are at greater risk; hence the importance of calling emergency services as soon as possible (see p. 41).

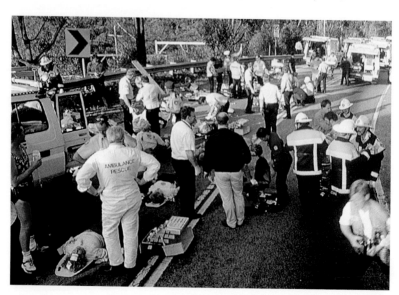

Disasters

In most cases where multiple casualties are involved, ambulance and hospital services are able to cope. However, in certain situations such as an earthquake, cyclone or major explosion, the number of casualties may exceed the capacity of the medical and rescue services. Because of the possibility of further casualties from secondary explosion and/or building collapse, and the need to minimise congestion, it is important to remove casualties from the accident site as soon as possible. In such an incident, the first aider may have to manage a team effort to give first aid to the casualties.

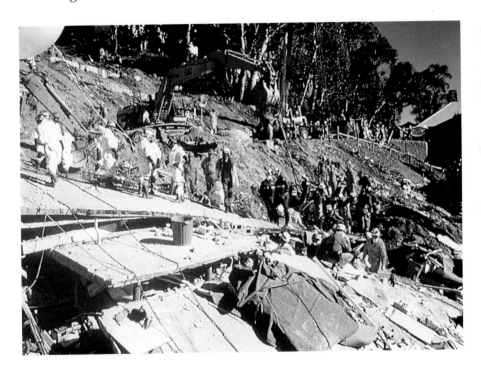

Triage with mass casualties

In an accident or disaster with mass casualties, the triage officer may have to make a choice between whom to save and whom to leave, possibly to die. This task is most appropriately performed by an experienced medical, nursing or ambulance practitioner.

In such a situation, the principles of triage remain the same. However, order of priority may be 'reversed'. Priority may be given to casualties whose injuries can be rapidly treated with a good chance of permanent recovery rather than to those whose injuries would be time-consuming to treat and probably result in significant permanent disability.

For example, a casualty with a fractured spine would generally have a lower priority than one with internal abdominal bleeding. The latter will probably fully recover with immediate hospital treatment but may die if treatment is left for an hour or so, whereas the former will probably result in permanent paralysis whether treatment is given straight away or in a few hours.

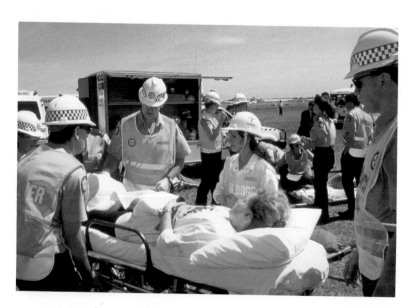

To decide the urgency of each casualty's need for care and evacuation, the first aider needs to be able to assess injuries according to a plan. In making such decisions, two main principles apply:

- Acute needs override long-term outcomes—a casualty with a fractured spine will generally have lower priority for evacuation than a casualty with internal abdominal bleeding.
- Life takes precedence over limb—a casualty who is not breathing has priority over a casualty who is bleeding providing the bleeding is not life-threatening. If the bleed is life-threatening, it should be treated first. However, as a general rule, airway management has the highest priority.

Site control centre

A site control centre should:

- be as near the accident site as possible
- be elevated so you can see the whole accident site
- be up wind
- be easily reached
- have communications available such as telephone and radio.

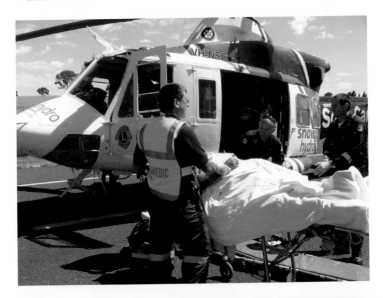

Triage areas should be distinctly marked and the site control centre well protected. It should be positioned so as to provide good access both to casualties and evacuation routes. As soon as practicable the first aider should hand over coordination to an emergency services or police officer. Usually the responding ambulance service will take charge of the care of casualties and will direct first aiders who may be able to stay at the scene and assist.

Ranking casualties

Triage specialists (ambulance paramedics) at a major accident site will rank (prioritise) casualties by attaching labels. For the first aider, the process is less formalised but the concept remains the same. It is important to remember that a casualty is always in a changing, not static, condition. This is especially important with head and abdominal injuries in which deterioration can occur.

Group 1

Casualties with minor injuries would not normally need medical treatment; (e.g. minor bruises or abrasions, fright, slight headache).

These casualties should be registered, then instructed by the police to leave the accident area unassisted or with a friend, to seek medical aid or return home.

Group 2

Casualties requiring medical treatment but not immediate hospitalisation; (e.g. ankle sprains, large bruises and abrasions, back strain).

These casualties can be evacuated to their homes after registration and instructed to seek early treatment from their own medical practitioner.

Note: Casualties classified in the preceding two groups should, if possible, receive appropriate first aid management prior to evacuation. However, they should not be allowed to crowd an accident site or delay attention to the more urgent cases. They are more likely to receive early medical treatment at home or at a private doctor's surgery than they are if transported to the hospital receiving the more seriously injured.

Group 3

Some casualties who require early transport to hospital will need urgent surgery to survive whereas others can wait.

This group can be further subdivided into priority cases:

Priority 1—require urgent transport to hospital

- breathing difficulties (e.g. flail chest, collapsed lung/lungs, obstructed airway)
- severe bleeding, abdominal injury with signs of shock, open fractures, crush injuries, or burns to 30% or more of body surface
- head injuries and deteriorating level of consciousness
- multiple injuries

Priority 2—may require surgery within a few hours

- unconscious with a clear airway
- abdominal injury without signs of shock
- large wounds where bleeding has been controlled
- burns to 10–30% of body surface
- fractures or dislocation of major joints

Priority 3—most will require surgery when practicable

- closed fractures
- facial injuries without airway obstruction
- eye injury
- minor wounds
- burns to less than 10% of body surface
- spinal injury

Group 4

Casualties clinically dead such as those who have been decapitated, and those who will probably die before reaching hospital, those who have massive head or torso injuries, whose brain and skull have been very severely damaged or who have been incinerated. These casualties are the last to be evacuated. They should be managed with dignity and protection.

The triage officer must not jeopardise the survival of those with a possibility of recovery by using ambulance and hospital resources for the untreatable because of fear of making an error.

25

First aid in a remote area

A remote area is defined as one where access to medical assistance is hampered by time and distance. This includes not only outback areas but also national parks, bushland, wilderness or mountain areas, and the sea. In any of these areas it may take some hours or even days to reach, or be reached by, emergency services.

Much of Australia is made up of remote and wilderness areas. The Australian outback, alpine wilderness and the many national parks all pose particular challenges to those dealing with an injured person. Knowing how to apply first aid and a readiness to be selfreliant will give confidence to all who live, work or travel in these areas.

Being able to manage injuries in a remote area in a skilled and confident manner may save a life. Help may be delayed— for a day or more—and transporting the injured to medical assistance can be a prolonged process. In such circumstances, skilled first aid can prevent complications and help with a speedy recovery.

Ideally, a walking party should consist of no less than 4 people. If a member of the group becomes injured it is safer if 2 members of the group go for help and the other person stays to care for the casualty. The general rule is that the most experienced first aider remains with the casualty.

Weather conditions, fires and floods can delay access to medical assistance. In remote areas medical, nursing and ambulance personnel are few in number and may be committed in other areas at the time of need. However, every effort should be made through the use of cellular or satellite telephones, or portable two-way radios, to establish a communication link to a medical facility. If you are able to establish a link, expert advice will be available, even in the most remote areas, to help you manage the casualty. This contact will also facilitate the pick up and transport of the casualty.

Management considerations

The principles of first aid are always the same, whether in remote areas or anywhere else. However, a sound knowledge of survival techniques and procedures for contacting medical assistance become especially important in remote areas.

Whether to continue an activity

The first aider will have to decide whether a casualty can continue with work or recreational activity or whether the activity should be abandoned to take the casualty to medical aid. The welfare of the group as a whole will also have to be considered in making these decisions.

Whether to travel to medical assistance or to wait for it to come

This will be influenced by such factors as the severity of the injury, time required for medical aid to arrive, risk that moving might hinder rescue efforts, whether the casualty can be moved safely, the safety of the location and the adequacy of food and water supplies.

Reassurance

The casualty can become more stressed because of the longer wait for medical assistance and may need greater emotional support and reassurance. Remaining calm and regularly monitoring the casualty's condition will help reduce both the casualty's and the first aider's anxieties.

The casualty's comfort

In remote locations there are going to be time delays before medical assistance arrives or evacuation can be implemented. It is important to ensure the casualty is comfortable until this can occur. The casualty's conscious state and nature of injuries will determine the most comfortable position.

Documentation

A first aider needs to be aware of the casualty's condition as this may change significantly during management. The first aider's observations and recording of changes are particularly significant—documenting everything (changes in signs and symptoms, vital signs, first aid management) is important and can be very helpful to medical staff in later treatment.

The need to monitor fluid intake and output

An important observation is the monitoring of fluids, irrespective of whether they are in a hot or cold environment. When a casualty evacuation or medical assistance is going to be delayed, the recording of fluid intake and output is important, especially to medical staff in the further management of the casualty.

Shelter and survival

There is a great need to ensure the casualty is sheltered from the elements. If in a cold climate, keep the casualty warm and dry with added clothing, blankets, paper or any other material that will help insulate the body. If in a hot climate, keep the casualty in the shade and out of direct sun, loosen clothing and wipe casualty with a wet cloth if possible. Do not forget to provide for your own shelter.

Shock

In most cases where a casualty has sustained an injury or has become seriously ill they may develop shock. The longer a sick or injured casualty remains without medical treatment, the greater the potential for shock. The management of the casualty is crucial in preventing the shock from developing further.

The need to perform a procedure for which you are not trained

In some cases you may have to perform a procedure which is beyond your training (e.g. an injection). In these types of situations you may be required to have medical supplies that are pertinent to your situation. With the assistance of telephone or radio instructions from emergency services, the Royal Flying Doctor Service or a medical practitioner will instruct you on how to perform these procedures.

Trauma management plan

Assess the situation – calling for medical assistance

By assessing the situation you are looking at what happened—for example, a fall of approximately five metres—is it reasonable to expect the casualty will be seriously injured? Can you see from where you are if the casualty is seriously injured—for example, is blood pouring out of several injuries? If the answer is yes, direct that emergency services be contacted.

If you believe the injuries are serious, do not hesitate to begin to get help as soon as the situation allows. Any delay in calling for help may affect the casualty's chance of survival.

Check for any danger

In the rush to assist the casualty, it is easy for danger to be overlooked. The first aider needs to quickly assess the scene for any danger to themselves. Certainly in the situation where someone is seriously injured time is of the essence, but rushing in without considering the risk to yourself and other rescuers may result in the situation becoming more desperate if a rescuer or another person is also injured.

Check that casualty can breathe effectively

If the casualty is conscious ask them,'Can you breathe all
right?' If the answer is yes, ask them to take a deep breath.
If the casualty cannot breathe effectively, check their chest for
injuries. A severely injured casualty with a chest injury, who
is breathless and can only breathe with some effort, or whose
breathing is hardly sufficient to cause the chest to rise, is best
managed by carefully rolling them on to their injured side. If
the casualty is unconscious they should be rolled onto their
side to maintain a clear and open airway.

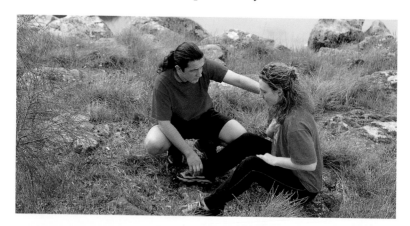

Stop bleeding

In remote areas a casualty who is bleeding heavily is at risk.
The bleeding must be stopped quickly. Shirts and towels, for
example, make effective pads to stop bleeding when held
firmly on a wound.

Stabilise head and neck

An injury to the neck should be suspected:
* when the unconscious casualty has a head injury
* when any casualty has a serious head injury
* in all velocity accidents—that is, when force has been
  involved, such as in falls.

While the priority is to manage life-threatening problems such as inability to breathe effectively and/or severe bleeding, the possibility of a neck injury must be considered and the casualty's neck stabilised as soon as possible. This can be achieved quickly and effectively by holding the casualty's head steady with your hands or using material to pack and maintain the position of the head and stop movement.

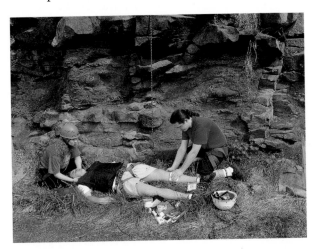

Check casualty for other injuries – head-to-toe assessment

It is important to quickly and thoroughly check the casualty from head to toe for other serious injuries. Small non-bleeding wounds and broken bones should not interfere with the process. They can be managed later. The priority is to ensure there are no other heavily bleeding wounds.

History

Much is made of obtaining a history from casualties concerning allergies, existing medical conditions, medications and so on. While this may be of value at a later time, it is not a priority when managing a seriously injured casualty. The aim is to keep them alive. The first aider must direct all their attention and skill to managing the injuries.

Once all injuries are managed and the casualty is protected, attention can then be given to collecting a medical history. As the immediate dangers have in part been addressed, ambulance and hospital staff will be able to devote time to gaining further information about the casualty's medical history. To assist with obtaining this information the acronym **AMPLE** should be applied:

Allergies—any allergies

Medication—taking any form of medication, e.g. anticoagulants

Past/present medical history—e.g. heart condition

Last meal/drink—when was the last meal and fluid intake

Event/environment—what happened, when, how did it happen, signs and symptoms, observations.

Managing a serious injury

1 Call Emergency Services/Ambulance

2 Check for danger

- advise casualty not to move.

3 Can casualty breathe ok?

- YES—stop visible bleeding

- NO—prioritise bleeding or breathing.

4 Stabilise head and neck

Note: If sufficient help available, neck may be stabilised earlier.

5 Head-to-toes assessment

- manage what is found, manage for shock.

6 History

- survival may depend on effective management of injuries

- do not interrupt management to obtain medical history.

Casualty care

Observing and recording the casualty's condition

In a remote area it may be necessary to observe a casualty for a prolonged time. The type of observations will be determined by the casualty's condition and injuries. For example, a simple lower limb fracture does not usually require you to note the level of consciousness, pulse, breathing and pupil changes. However, it could be vital to observe and record colour and condition of the toes on the injured limb.

Remember that a casualty's condition can deteriorate. Close observation of the casualty will help early recognition of any changes and assist in further management. The recording and transmitting of such changes are of great help to rescue services.

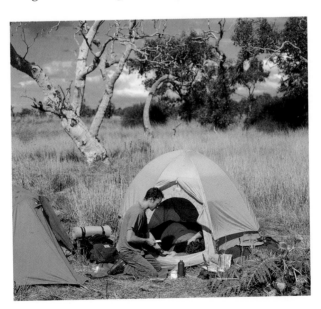

It is particularly important to record initial observations. For a severely injured casualty, observations should be made every 15 minutes; for a less seriously injured casualty, observations may be made at half hourly to hourly intervals.

Observe and regularly record the casualty's:

- **conscious state—especially time of any changes:**
  - has it improved or deteriorated?
- **pulse—count rate over 1 minute and record:**
  - is rate fast or slow?
  - is rhythm regular or irregular?
  - is it weak or strong?
- **breathing—count rate over 1 minute and record:**
  - is rate fast or slow?
  - is it deep, shallow or sighing?
  - is it noisy, quiet or gurgling?
- **temperature—especially any changes:**
  - is it normal?
  - is it above/below 37°C?
- **pupils—especially time of any changes:**
  - are they dilated or contracted?
  - are they equal or unequal?
  - do they react to light?
- **skin colour:**
  - is it normal or pale?
  - is it bluish or purplish?
- **skin condition:**
  - is it wet or dry?
  - is it warm or cold?
- **speech:**
  - is it slurred?
- **fluid intake and output** (*see p. 473*).

Take care if discussing casualty—don't assume the casualty cannot hear or understand you even if apparently unconscious.

Managing illnesses and injuries

In a remote area, control of blood loss and infection can be more demanding because blood loss may continue over a long time. Management may need to be modified depending on supplies on hand. For example, the number of dressings available will dictate the number of dressing changes.

A first aider will also have to decide the seriousness of an injury to determine how urgently medical assistance is required. Is there damage to underlying body structures? How much damage is there? What level of shock is likely?

All wounds can become infected. When dirt and debris enter and remain in penetrating or deep wounds, infection always occurs. Such wounds need to be attended to urgently. Superficial wounds can also become infected. Abrasions can be dangerous when they involve large areas of the body, because of the risk of infection and shock. Ensure any wound is kept clean and, if wound is open, cover with a dressing. An infected wound is painful, debilitating and prolongs recovery. In warm and humid climates, a casualty who suffers a wound is at a much greater risk of infection, particularly if medical aid is delayed.

Checking adequacy of dressings, bandages and splints

1 Inspect the dressings to see if blood has soaked through:

- add further dressings if necessary

- make sure dressings are sufficiently tight.

2 Check any fracture immobilisation for firmness of bandages:

- if loosened, apply a firm bandage over initial bandage.

3 Check circulation of limb:

- if fingers or toes are pale, painful, or cold and numb, remove bandage and re-apply.

Moving a casualty

In remote areas a seriously injured casualty should not be moved unless necessary. The casualty must be moved if:

- in danger from storms, lightning, flood or fire
- you decide the benefits outweigh the destabilisation that movement might produce.

Local movement may be needed for comfort, but there may be snakes, ants or other creatures that could create further problems. There may be discomfort or fear, or the ground may be cold, or the place where the accident occurred could be dangerous (e.g. on a narrow ledge), uncomfortable, exposed or inaccessible.

It is not recommended, but if you have to transport the casualty in a private vehicle, it is important to remain calm, and to drive at a safe speed. No matter how serious the injury or the circumstances, excessive speed will only endanger yourself and the casualty, and aggravate injuries.

Improvisation

The ability to improvise and to use whatever resources are available is a valuable skill for the first aider.

Clothing and other items may be used to control bleeding, to tie and support fractures and to pad injured parts of the body:

- Tea towels, socks, pillowcases, a sheet or torn piece of clothing can control bleeding or be used as dressings.
- Singlets, folded shirts, blouses and trousers can make padding or, if twisted tightly round and round, a ring pad around a foreign object.
- Shoelaces can tie padding to a splint.
- Shirts, singlets and blouses can be cut into strips for roller bandages.
- Long socks, long sleeves or clothing cut into 20 cm strips can make collar and cuff slings.
- Coats and jackets with poles passed through sleeves can make stretchers.

Other items can also be used—sacks and sleeping bags with poles passed through them can be used as stretchers, as can flat pieces of strong material (e.g. lengths of timber, door, side panel of a vehicle); tree branches can be used as splints or poles; folded newspaper can be used as a splint.

Toiletting hygiene and comfort

The mobile casualty can use a latrine dug in the ground. However, if the casualty is not mobile, a billy can, water bottle, plastic bag or other container can be used as an improvised urinal.

For bowel motions, a large plastic bag is suitable. It is essential the casualty's hands are washed after toiletting, and that waste is buried in a deep pit, at least 60 cm deep to prevent the waste from being dug up by fauna. Handwashing and infection control procedures (standard precautions) should be followed whenever possible (see p.133).

Fluid intake and output

When evacuation may be delayed for some time, it is necessary to ensure the casualty maintains an adequate fluid intake to prevent dehydration. However, the amount of fluid given will be determined by the type and extent of the casualty's injuries and level of consciousness. Casualties not severely injured may eat and drink as usual. But if a casualty shows signs and symptoms of shock, and if you are more than three hours from help, you should give clear fluids if the casualty can take them. If the casualty, especially a child, has diarrhoea, give as much fluid as the casualty wants. Frequent small amounts are best. Energy drinks are ideal and should be carried by all who venture into the outback and other remote areas.

Casualties who have abdominal pain, a reduced level of consciousness or who cannot pass urine should not usually be given any fluids, or only sips at the most. However, mouth and lip care are important—wipe face and lips and apply lanolin cream as lip balm if available.

For other casualties:

- moisten casualty's lips with water for the first 4–8 hours after injury
- give small amounts of water (e.g. 100 ml/half a cup) every half hour if medical aid has not arrived after 4–8 hours— consider increasing the quantity in hotter climates
- stop giving water if the casualty vomits or shows other signs of discomfort
- if surgical care is likely within 4–6 hours, do not give food or drink to a casualty whose condition is serious— for example, severe open fractures, internal injuries, and fractures that involve other organs (e.g. skull and pelvic fractures).

It is necessary to monitor fluid intake and output when the casualty:

- drinks water
- vomits
- passes urine
- loses blood
- develops diarrhoea.

Where possible, the volume should be recorded using a convenient measure such as a cup or soup tin. The measuring device should be kept with the casualty and shown to medical personnel. Blood, vomit, faeces and excessive sweating can be difficult to measure and may simply be recorded as being 'small', 'moderate' or 'large'. The time should also be recorded. Note whether urine is concentrated or odourless and whether blood (smokiness) is present.

General nursing care

A casualty who lies immobile for long periods of time may develop reddened pressure areas over bony prominences such as heels, buttocks, and shoulderblades. Facial areas such as ears are of particular concern. Circulation becomes impaired to skin areas that remain in contact with hard surfaces such as the ground. These skin areas need to be relieved of pressure by using padding and turning the casualty every 2 hours. Turn more frequently if skin becomes damaged and a sore develops. Care for all unconscious casualties in the recovery position.

26

How the body functions

The body's systems

The body is made up of systems which have different functions to perform in keeping the body alive and well. Each system has a function to perform, but none works independently.

This chapter outlines the functions of each system and the role of the major associated organs. The skeleton, which is the body's supporting structure, is also described.

Circulatory system

The circulatory system comprises the heart, blood and blood vessels (veins, arteries and capillaries). It keeps all parts of the body supplied with oxygen-rich blood and the various sugars, proteins, vitamins, minerals and hormones needed for growth and health. This system also transports carbon dioxide, urea and other waste products to be eliminated.

Respiratory system

The respiratory system includes the lungs, windpipe or trachea (airway from larynx to lungs), bronchi (two tubes branching off the trachea), bronchioles (smaller tubes branching off the bronchi), millions of alveoli (air sacs), and diaphragm (a smooth flat muscle under the lungs). This system keeps the body supplied with oxygen and removes carbon dioxide.

Digestive and urinary system

The digestive and urinary systems are made up of the oesophagus (gullet), stomach, liver, kidneys, gall bladder, pancreas, small and large intestines, rectum, bladder and urethra. These systems have two main functions: to convert food to simpler substances and a finer consistency so it can be absorbed into the blood and taken to all parts of the body; and to eliminate waste products.

Nervous system

The nervous system includes the brain, the spinal cord and the network of nerves which go to every part of the body. This system transports information from one part of the body to another, using electrical impulses and chemicals.

Lymphatic system

The lymphatic system includes lymph, lymph vessels, lymph nodes and the spleen. It is responsible for transporting lymph, a fluid containing white cells used in the fight against infection.

Musculoskeletal system

The musculoskeletal system consists of the bones, muscles, ligaments and tendons which support the body, protect the internal organs and allow the various parts of the body to move.

Body systems—in summary

System	Major organs	Major functions
Circulatory	heart, blood, blood vessels	• transports nutrients and oxygen • removes waste products
Respiratory	airway, lungs	• supplies oxygen • removes waste gases
Digestive and urinary	stomach, intestines, pancreas, rectum, kidneys, bladder, urethra	• converts food and liquids into proteins, sugars and other substances • collects and eliminates waste products
Nervous	brain, spinal cord, nerves	• transmits messages to and from brain
Lymphatic	lymph, lymph nodes, spleen	• fights infection
Musculoskeletal	bones, ligaments, muscles, tendon	• provides body's framework • protects internal organs • provides the mechanical basis for movement

Circulatory system

The circulatory system is a complex circuit which enables blood to circulate throughout the entire body, transporting oxygen and nutrients to every cell and collecting waste products for elimination from the body.

The heart provides the pumping action needed to keep blood flowing throughout the body. The heart is a muscular organ the size of a clenched fist which acts as a two-sided pump, first relaxing and filling up with blood and then contracting to squeeze (or pump) the blood out into the arteries. This pumping action is automatic and is controlled by a complex system of nerves.

Blood

Blood is made up of:

- plasma—pale yellow liquid in which blood cells are suspended; contains proteins, electrolytes and various nutrients; is capable of clotting
- red blood cells—carry oxygen
- white blood cells—protect body from germs
- platelets—form clots to stop bleeding.

Pulse

The heart's contractions can be felt in the arteries close to the skin, primarily at the neck (carotid artery), wrist (radial artery) and groin (femoral artery). The beat felt with each contraction is called a pulse.

Blood vessels

Arteries are large, strong blood vessels which carry oxygen-rich blood to all parts of the body. They subdivide into smaller blood vessels then capillaries—tiny, thin-walled blood vessels which transport blood to all cells of the body. After the cells receive oxygen from the blood, veins carry the blood, now low in oxygen, to the heart and then to the lungs.

Circulation

The circulation of blood begins and ends at the heart and consists of:

- pulmonary circulation—starting on the right side of the heart, blood is pumped to the lungs where it loses carbon dioxide and absorbs oxygen, and then goes back to the left side of the heart

- systemic circulation—starting on the left side of the heart, blood is pumped to the body, where it delivers oxygen and removes carbon dioxide, and then returns to the right side of the heart.

Effects of bleeding

If an injury results in external or internal bleeding, the body tries to minimise blood loss. When a blood vessel is damaged, it will contract to slow or stop blood loss through the wound, and clots form to further restrict the bleeding. If bleeding is heavy, the contraction of blood vessels also helps to maintain blood pressure. With continued blood loss, the body has trouble compensating and blood pressure drops. The casualty then starts showing signs of shock.

Body tissues that do not receive enough oxygen can be permanently damaged or die. If an artery supplying the brain is blocked, brain cells die, resulting in a stroke. A heart attack occurs when an artery supplying the heart with blood is blocked. Some muscle cells die, leading to damaged heart muscle.

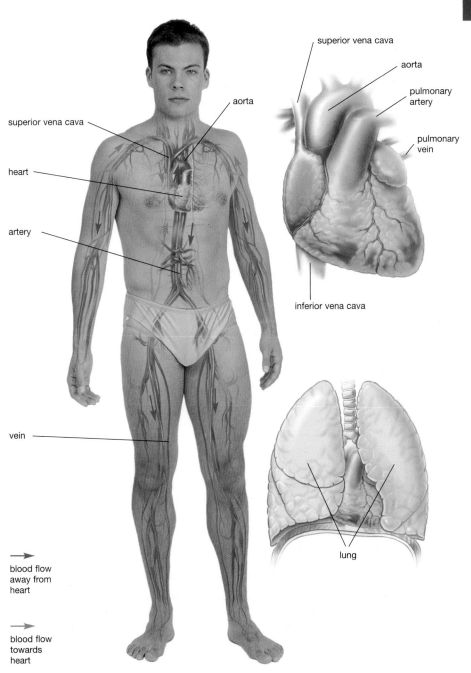

superior vena cava

aorta

aorta

superior vena cava

pulmonary artery

heart

pulmonary vein

artery

inferior vena cava

vein

lung

blood flow away from heart

blood flow towards heart

Respiratory system

The body needs a constant supply of oxygen to function and survive. When a person inhales, air is taken into the air sacs of the lungs where oxygen crosses to the blood to be transported to all parts of the body. The blood also brings carbon dioxide and other waste gases from around the body to the lungs where it crosses to the air sacs. This waste is then forced from the body when a person exhales. Inhaled air contains 21% oxygen while exhaled air contains about 16% oxygen and more carbon dioxide than inhaled air. (The 16% oxygen in exhaled breath is sufficient to give to a non-breathing casualty during CPR.)

Mechanics of breathing

The diaphragm and the muscles between the ribs (intercostals), work together to expand the chest. When the chest expands, air is pulled into the lungs. As these muscles relax, the chest returns to its usual size and the air is forced out. Using extra muscles in the neck and shoulders can increase the force and rate of breathing. These are used in exercise or when a person is suffering from chest disease.

Inhalation

Air is breathed in through the mouth or nose and passes down the trachea to the two bronchi which take the air into the lungs. The bronchi then branch further into a number of smaller tubes called bronchioles which end in millions of tiny air sacs called alveoli. The walls of the alveoli and capillaries are thin so that oxygen and carbon dioxide cross through them. Thus oxygen enters the blood and carbon dioxide enters the alveoli.

Oxygen–carbon dioxide balance

The part of the brain which controls respiration monitors the amount of oxygen and carbon dioxide in the blood and responds to changes in these levels by changing the rate and depth of breathing. The amount of oxygen being used by the body is related to the amount of physical activity. The more energetic the activity, the greater the amount of oxygen required and the more carbon dioxide produced. Fever and illness may also increase demands for oxygen.

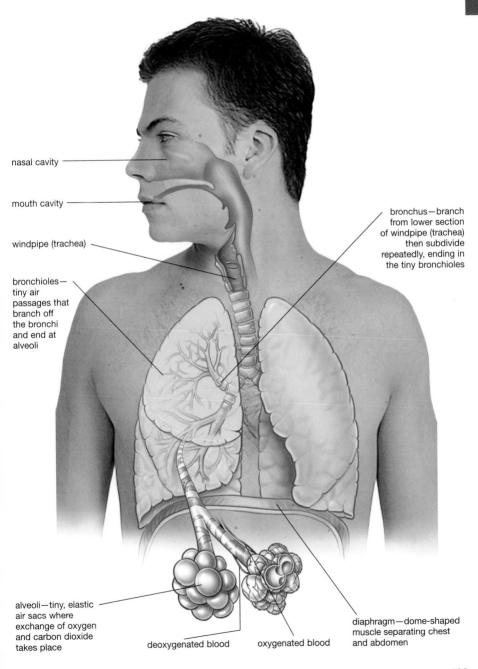

nasal cavity

mouth cavity

windpipe (trachea)

bronchioles—
tiny air
passages that
branch off
the bronchi
and end at
alveoli

bronchus—branch
from lower section
of windpipe (trachea)
then subdivide
repeatedly, ending in
the tiny bronchioles

alveoli—tiny, elastic
air sacs where
exchange of oxygen
and carbon dioxide
takes place

deoxygenated blood

oxygenated blood

diaphragm—dome-shaped
muscle separating chest
and abdomen

Digestive and urinary systems

The digestive system converts food and liquid into nutrients
to keep the cells functioning. It also removes waste products.

Food moves from the mouth, where saliva has begun the
process of breaking the food down, through the oesophagus
to the stomach where it is partly digested by gastric juices.
As the food is expelled from the stomach it is mixed with
other digestive juices from the pancreas (insulin), liver and
gall bladder. These juices help to break down the complex
structure of the food into simpler forms. Insulin helps
control blood sugar levels.

The food then moves on to the small intestine where the
digestive process is completed and the nutrients are absorbed
into the blood. The material left after this process moves to
the large intestine and is eliminated from the rectum as faeces.

Urinary system

Other waste products are extracted from the blood by the
kidneys which produce between one and two litres of urine
daily. This moves down the ureter to the bladder, where it is
held until it is voided through the urethra.

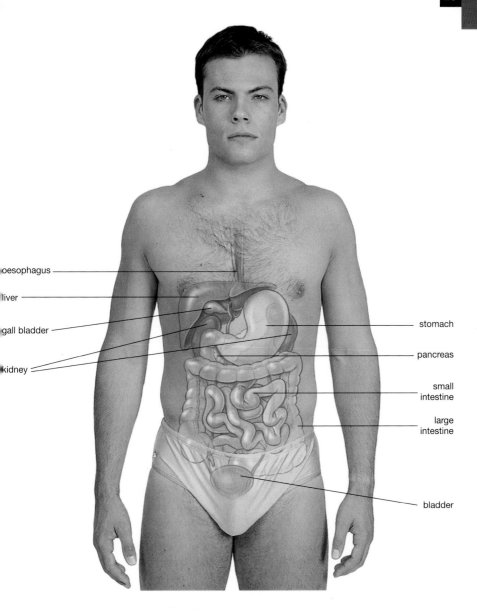

oesophagus

liver

gall bladder

kidney

stomach

pancreas

small intestine

large intestine

bladder

Nervous system

The nervous system is made up of the brain, spinal cord and nerves.

Brain

The brain is the controlling organ of the body and regulates all body functions. Through the body's network of nerves, the brain receives and transmits information as electrical impulses and chemicals.

Sensory and motor nerves

Sensory nerves, which transmit impulses from the body to the brain, relay information about touch, sight, sound, smell, taste, spatial awareness and pain. Motor nerves control movement by initiating muscle contraction.

Spinal cord

The spinal cord is a large group of nerves which extends from the brain down the backbone through a canal in the spine. Nerves extend from the brain and the spinal cord to every part of the body. At each vertebra of the spinal cord, two nerves branch out, one to each side of the body. In the upper part of the spinal cord, just below the brain, are the autonomic centres for breathing and heart control.

Voluntary and autonomic systems

The voluntary nervous system controls the functions directed by the conscious mind, (e.g. walking, running and eating). The autonomic nervous system controls involuntary functions such as heartbeat, breathing, digestion and blood pressure.

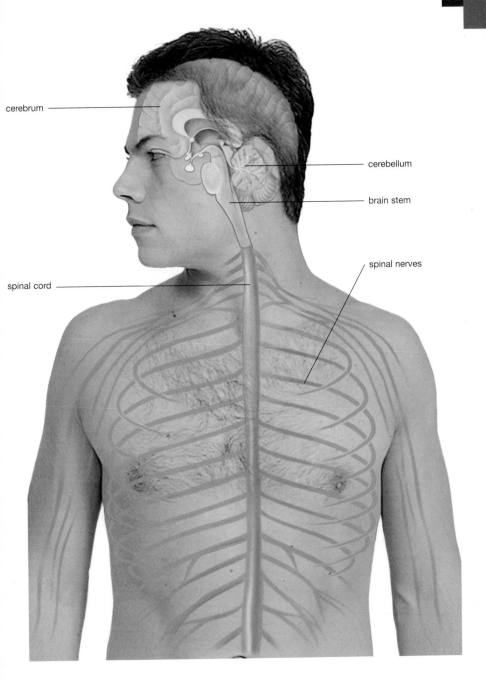

cerebrum

cerebellum

brain stem

spinal nerves

spinal cord

Lymphatic system

The lymphatic vessels pick up fluid that has been left behind in the tissues by the circulatory system and transports it back to the main veins just before they reach the heart. The lymphatic vessels come from all over the body. They contain one-way valves so that the fluid they carry flows only towards the heart. This fluid (lymph) contains white blood cells, giving the lymphatic system a role in fighting infection.

Lymph nodes

As lymph fluid is transported towards the heart, it passes through lymph nodes (sometimes referred to as glands), which contain many white cells and serve as filters. The white cells form antibodies and remove bacteria, viruses and other foreign substances. When they become activated, lymph nodes will sometimes become enlarged. This can occur before and during many common infections (e.g. influenza, glandular fever, septicaemia and skin infections). Lymph nodes may be felt in the neck, under the arm and in the groin.

White cells and spleen

White cells are found throughout the body. As well as producing antibodies and fighting infection, they have a role to play in removing and repairing old tissue, in causing fever, and in inflammation and repair of wounds. The spleen carries out these functions, as well as being a filter for the blood, and has the body's biggest concentration of white cells.

The importance of the immunity given by white blood cells is seen in conditions like AIDS, in which the white cells are destroyed slowly by the human immunodeficiency virus (HIV) and the body becomes susceptible to many infections that would not normally cause illness.

Lymph vessels and toxins

The lymphatic vessels provide the major route by which many venomous toxins enter the circulatory system. By using the pressure immobilisation bandage and keeping a limb still by splinting, it is possible to slow or even stop lymph fluid entering the circulation.

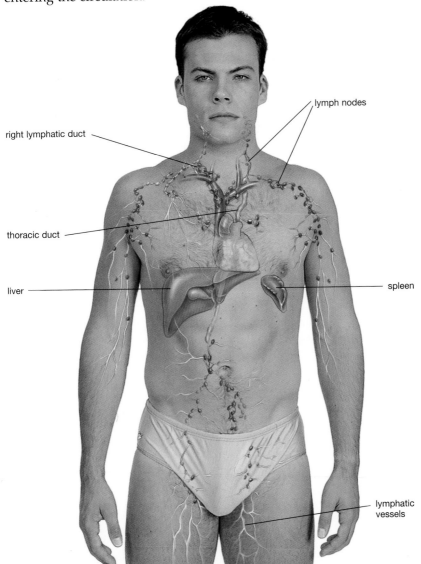

lymph nodes

right lymphatic duct

thoracic duct

liver

spleen

lymphatic vessels

Musculoskeletal system

The musculoskeletal system is made up of various bones, muscles, tendons, ligaments and joints. It provides support for the body, gives protection to internal organs, stores minerals, produces blood cells in the marrow and makes movement possible.

The skeleton is the supporting structure that gives the body its general shape and provides a strong framework to which muscles are attached. It also protects many of the organs such as the brain which is protected by the skull, the heart and lungs by the rib cage, and the spinal cord by the vertebrae of the spine.

Bones

The bones which make up the skeleton are dense, very strong structures that have an ample supply of blood and nerves. Some bones store and manufacture red blood cells in the marrow.

Joints

Joints are held together by ligaments and are found wherever bones meet. There are two types of joints: movable and immovable. Immovable joints are fused (e.g. the skull). Some movable joints allow slight movement (e.g. vertebrae). Others allow more movement (e.g. ball-and-socket joint of shoulder).

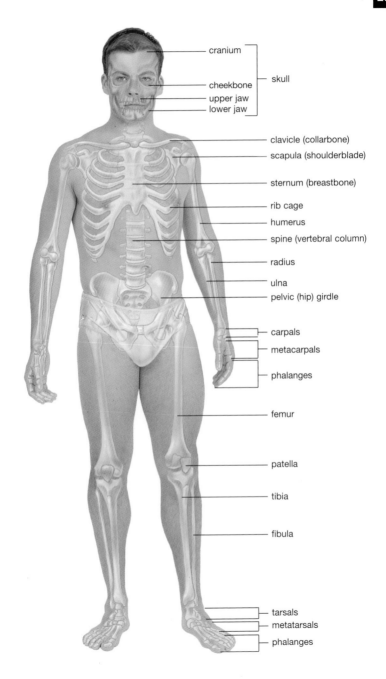

cranium

cheekbone

skull

upper jaw

lower jaw

clavicle (collarbone)

scapula (shoulderblade)

sternum (breastbone)

rib cage

humerus

spine (vertebral column)

radius

ulna

pelvic (hip) girdle

carpals

metacarpals

phalanges

femur

patella

tibia

fibula

tarsals

metatarsals

phalanges

Muscles and tendons

Muscles are mostly (but not all) attached to bones by strong fibrous tissue called tendons. Muscles account for up to 50% of a person's body weight. By contracting and relaxing, muscles move the bones, causing the limbs and digits to move.

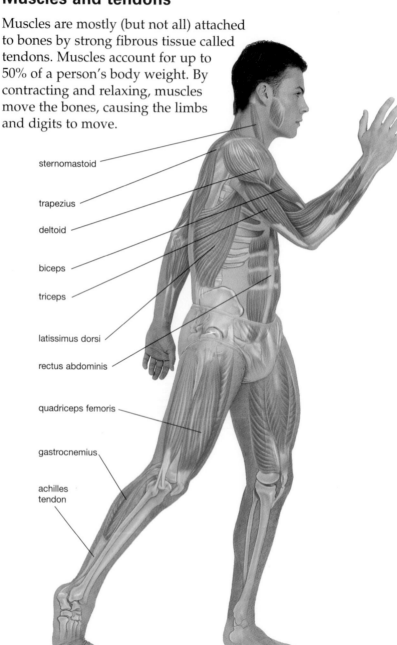

sternomastoid

trapezius

deltoid

biceps

triceps

latissimus dorsi

rectus abdominis

quadriceps femoris

gastrocnemius

achilles tendon

Glossary

Abdomen part of the body between chest and pelvis, containing digestive organs

Abrasion an open wound caused by direct contact with a rough surface

Acetone a colourless liquid used as a solvent (smells like nail polish remover)

Acid a corrosive substance; a neutraliser of an alkali

Acute pain a pain which is sharp, of sudden onset, severe and short in duration

Afterbirth the placenta, cord and membranes expelled after delivery of baby

AIDS acquired immune deficiency syndrome; condition causing serious illness and death through breakdown in functioning of body's immune system (see also HIV)

Airway the passage, starting at mouth or nose, through which air enters and leaves the lungs

Alkali a corrosive substance; a neutraliser of acid

Allergic sensitive to some substance foreign to the body, such as bee venom or certain foods

Alveoli air sacs in the lungs

Amputation cutting off of a limb, digit, or appendage

Anaphylactic shock an extreme and generalised allergic reaction

Angina a heart condition involving acute pain or angina pectoris—unpleasant sensation in chest caused by interference with supply of oxygen to heart, usually brought on by exercise or anxiety

Antiseptic a substance that kills germs or helps to prevent their growth

Anus the external opening of the rectum

Apex pulse heartbeat felt in newborn baby, in chest below left nipple

Arterial tourniquet device used to restrict the blood supply to a limb

Artery a vessel through which oxygen-bearing blood is pumped away from the heart

Asphyxia blockage of oxygen supply entering the lungs

Aspirate suck out using a suction device

Assessment evaluation of problems affecting casualty as indicated by history, symptoms and signs observed by first aider

Asthma spasm of bronchial (breathing) tubes in the lungs

Atherosclerosis narrowing of the arteries

Autonomic nervous system the branch of the nervous system that regulates unconscious   bodily functions (e.g. sweating)

Avulsion a wound in which skin is partially or completely torn away

Bladder a sac acting as a reservoir, e.g. urinary bladder (for urine), gall bladder (for bile)

Blood pressure the force exerted by blood against walls of blood vessels

Bone marrow soft interior of bones in which cells are produced

Bowel part of digestive canal below stomach and duodenum

BPC dressing standard British Pharmaceutical Codex dressing

Brachial pulse heartbeat felt on inner upper arm (usually used for infants)

Breastbone (also called sternum) flat bone which forms middle of front of chest and helps separate and support ribs

Bronchi large air passages that divide from windpipe

Capillaries smallest blood vessels

Carbon dioxide a gas which is part of the air we breathe out; waste product of human metabolism

Cardiac relating to the heart

Cardiopulmonary resuscitation also called CPR—resuscitation technique that combines rescue breaths with external cardiac compression

Carotid pulse heartbeat felt on arteries of neck

Casualty a person, alive or dead, who has suffered an accident or sudden illness

Cells the 'building blocks', microscopic in size, which in their countless millions make up the body

Cerebral relating to the brain

Cervical relating to the neck

Cholesterol fatty substance which circulates in blood and may be deposited into walls of arteries

Circulation movement of blood through the body

Coccyx tail bone—lowest part of spine

Compress used to supply cold to reduce bruising, swelling, and help relieve pain

Concussion any injury to the brain, usually caused by a blow, which leads to an altered state of consciousness or to unconsciousness

Constrictive bandage a firmly applied bandage used to control movement of tissue fluid or blood in a limb

Contusion a bruise or closed wound caused by a blow from a blunt object

Convulsions (also called seizures or fits) violent and involuntary contractions of limbs and body, accompanied by loss of consciousness

Corked thigh bruised thigh, with spasm

Cornea clear tissue in front of eye

Corrosive capable of destroying tissue by eating away a surface

CPR cardiopulmonary resuscitation

Cranium skeleton of head, excluding face and jaws

Crater wound caused by tissue being torn from the body

Cyanosis bluish discoloration of the skin and mucous membranes

Defibrillation application of a controlled electric shock to restore heart rhythm to normal

Dehydration excessive loss of water from the body

Diabetes disease caused by loss of insulin-producing cells in pancreas

Diaphragm dome-shaped muscular wall separating abdomen from chest cavity

Diarrhoea overly frequent and soft or liquid bowel motions

Digestive glands the salivary glands, liver, gall bladder and pancreas

Disc a layer of fibro-elastic tissue between the vertebrae

Dislocation injury in which bones of a joint are pushed out of normal contact with each other

Disorientation a state of mental confusion, particularly relating to time and place

Distend swell out, inflate

DRABCD stands for Danger, Response, Airway, Breathing, CPR, Defibrillation—the St John action plan for first aid management

Dressing material used to cover a wound

Drug any substance, natural or artificial, causing some specific or abnormal physical or mental change

Emphysema a chronic condition of the lungs which causes severe restriction of breathing

Envenomation poisoning which results from injection of a venom from bites, stings or penetrating wounds inflicted by reptiles, insects and marine creatures

495

Epilepsy a condition of the brain leading to seizures or altered conscious states

EpiPen® auto injector device that delivers a metered dose of adrenaline

External cardiac compressions rhythmic compression of heart from outside the body; pressing on breastbone to provide artificial circulation of blood; also known as ECC

Extremities fingers and toes

Faeces waste food products passed by the bowel

Fainting a reversible form of loss of consciousness, due to a sudden insufficiency in supply of blood to the brain

Febrile convulsion (see Infantile convulsion)

Fibrillation (see Ventricular fibrillation)

Flail chest a condition caused by multiple fractures of ribs and instability of rib cage

Fracture a break in a bone

Gall bladder a sac in the upper abdomen which stores bile

Gastroenteritis inflammation of the stomach and intestine, leading to vomiting and/or diarrhoea

Genitals the external reproductive organs

Glands organs that secrete specific substances

Gullet (or oesophagus) the passage from back of throat to stomach

Haematoma an accumulation of blood leaked into tissues from damaged blood vessels resulting from an injury such as a blow

Hallucinations perception of imaginary sights and sounds

Hallucinogen a drug that causes hallucinations

Heart the hollow muscular organ responsible for pumping blood

Heatstroke a serious, life-threatening condition in which body temperature is dangerously high

History when relating to first aid, story of incident or illness, obtained from casualty or witnesses

HIV human immunodeficiency virus—causes clinical illness called AIDS

Hyperextend extend beyond normal position

Hyperglycaemia high blood sugar

Hypertension high blood pressure

Hyperthermia excessive heating of the body

Hyperventilation involuntary overbreathing which disturbs the oxygen–carbon dioxide balance in the blood

Hypoglycaemia low blood sugar

Hypothermia excessive cooling of the body, usually accidental and often serious

Hypoxia inadequate oxygen at the cellular level

Immobilise to prevent from moving

Incision a cut made by a sharp object

Inebriated drunk

Infantile convulsion caused by rapid rise in temperature in infants and young children (also called febrile convulsion; can also occur in adults)

Infection the invasion and growth of harmful germs in tissues and fluids of body

Infectious disease caused by germs such as bacteria and viruses that can spread from one person to another

Inflammation an abnormal state of the tissues characterised by pain, heat, swelling and redness

Insulin a hormone produced in the pancreas which controls level of sugar in blood and body cells

Intestines lower part of alimentary canal

Intoxication a state of excitement, altered conscious state or coma, induced by alcohol or other drugs

Irrigate to wash a wound with a constant stream of water or other fluid

Irukandji a very small stinging jellyfish found in tropical waters of Australia

Jimble small jellyfish most common in coastal waters of South Australia

Laceration a break in skin made by tearing or cutting

Larynx voice box

Lethal deadly

Ligaments tissues connecting or supporting bones at joints

Liver a large organ located in upper abdomen with an important filtering role in digestion; produces bile; metabolises fat etc.

Lungs the pair of breathing organs in the chest cavity

Mallet finger injury to end joint of finger

Medic Alert® bracelet worn to indicate a medical condition

Medication medicine in any form—liquid, tablet, inhalation or injection

Micro-organism a microscopic organism, e.g. germs, virus

Mucus sticky fluid from some parts of body, e.g. nose, bronchi

Nausea a feeling of sickness with possible vomiting

Neonatal newborn or in first four weeks of life

Nerves fibres that convey impulses from one part of the body to another

Organ a body part consisting of tissues grouped together to perform a specific function

Oropharyngeal relating to the passage that extends from mouth and nasal cavity down to upper end of gullet and windpipe

Oropharyngeal airway a device used to assist in establishing and maintaining an adequate airway

Oropharyngeal aspiration sucking fluid from mouth and nose to prevent inhalation of fluid, and to obtain and maintain an unobstructed airway

Oxygen a life-sustaining gaseous element of air

Pallor paleness of skin

Pancreas a gland that produces insulin and alkaline digestive matter

Paradoxical breathing seen in flail chest injuries—the injured side moves in on inhalation and balloons out on exhalation, instead of, as normal, the other way round

Paralysis inability to move parts of the body

Paraplegic paralysed from the waist down

Pelvis the bone structure that forms lowest part of trunk

Perineum pelvic area between genitals and anus

Placenta special tissue attached to mother's uterus, from which unborn baby is nourished and from which umbilical cord emerges

Plasma fluid component of blood

Platelets microscopic cells which float in blood and are involved in the clotting process

Pneumothorax air in chest cavity but outside lung, causing collapse of lung

Post-traumatic occurring after a traumatic experience

Pressure pad firm pad applied over dressing to assist in control of bleeding

Puffer (or inhaler) device to deliver a regulated dose of asthma medication

Pulmonary relating to lungs

Pulse transmission of heartbeat felt in various parts of the body

Pupil opening in centre of iris (coloured part) of eye

Quadriplegic paralysed from the neck down

Radial pulse heartbeat felt beside crease lines of wrist, on same side as thumb

Rectum final section of alimentary canal ending in the anus

Red cells microscopic discs which float in the plasma of the blood and carry oxygen and carbon dioxide

Respiration breathing

Response a casualty's reply to a first aider squeezing a casualty's shoulders, enabling assessment of casualty's state of consciousness

Resuscitation attempt to revive a casualty who is unconscious and not breathing

RICE stands for Rest, Ice, Compression, Elevation—method used by first aiders to manage soft tissue injuries

Sacrum solid bony mass at base of spine which supports pelvis

Scrotum soft pouch hanging from below base of penis, containing the testes

Sedative a drug to calm the nerves

Seizures (sometimes called fits or convulsions) violent muscular contractions with loss of consciousness

Shock a condition in which the circulatory system is not carrying sufficient blood to the tissues

Shoulderblade flat bone of back, jointed with bone of upper arm

Side-effects unintended effects of taking a drug or medicine

Signs features of casualty's condition that can be seen, felt, heard or smelt

Sinus any of the eight cavities in the skull that are connected with the nasal cavity

Spacer device to improve delivery of asthma medication by a puffer/inhaler

Spasm sudden involuntary muscular contraction

Spinal cord the bundle of nerve tissue extending from base of brain to lower back; surrounded and protected by spine

Spleen an organ in the abdomen; helps fight infection

Splint rigid material used to immobilise a limb in treating fractures, dislocations or venomous bites or stings

Sprain stretching of ligaments beyond their normal range

Sputum mucus from lungs, bronchi and throat that is coughed up or spat out

Sterile free of germs

Sternum breastbone

Stoma artificial opening on body's surface, connecting to a surgically implanted tube (e.g. neck stoma for breathing)

Strain overstretching or overexertion of a muscle

Stroke a condition resulting from a blockage in blood supply to the brain, often involving partial paralysis and loss of speech

Suicide taking one's own life

Suffocation death from lack of oxygen

Symptoms what the casualty tells you about his or her condition

Testicles the male sex glands located in the scrotum

Tetanus a serious and potentially fatal infection, characterised by muscle spasms

Tissue a group of human body cells that performs a specific function

Toxic poisonous

Trachea windpipe

Trauma a wound, injury or other shocking experience

Triage classification and sorting of casualties for management and evacuation, according to degree of urgency

Umbilical cord the cord attaching unborn baby to placenta in mother's womb

Ureter tube leading from each kidney to bladder

Urine fluid containing waste products removed from blood by kidneys

Vagina passage leading inwards from external female genitalia

Varicose veins swollen veins, usually on the legs

Veins vessels that carry blood towards the heart

Venom a toxin (i.e. a poison made by a living thing), usually from a snake, insect, spider or marine creature; secreted and injected by bite or sting

Ventricular fibrillation a chaotic condition of the electrical impulses of the heart, interfering with normal beating

Vertebrae (singular: vertebra) bones that make up the spinal column

Vital signs physical signs of life including breathing, heartbeat and conscious state

Voice box (or larynx) part of windpipe where vocal cords are situated

Vomitus stomach contents projected from the stomach

Vulva external female genitals

White cells blood cells which float in plasma and combat infection

Windpipe (or trachea) air tube between throat and lungs

Index